# The Arthritis Handbook

*The Essential Guide to a Pain-Free, Drug-Free Life*

Grant Cooper, MD

Departments of Rehabilitation Medicine and Orthopedic Surgery
Beth Israel Medical Center, New York, New York

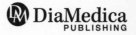

DiaMedica Publishing, 150 East 61st Street, New York, NY 10065

Visit our website at www.diamedicapub.com.

Library of Congress Cataloging-in-Publication Data available from the publisher upon request.

ISBN-13: 978-0-9793564-1-4
ISBN-10: 0-9793564-1-5

Note to Readers
This book is not a substitute for medical advice and assistance. The judgment of individual physicians and therapists who know you is essential. Although the information in this book was developed to help you manage your arthritis, it is not intended to replace your own physician's medical advice.

Editor: Jessica Bryan
Designed and typeset by: Gopa & Ted 2, Inc.
Printed in Canada

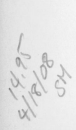

# Contents

# Acknowledgments

THANK YOU to my wife, Ana, for being my daily source of strength, laughter, and inspiration. In addition, Ana has lent her medical and literary expertise to help read and revise many pages in this book. She has served as the sounding board for many of my ideas, and she is also the beautiful model who demonstrates the exercises. Writing this book has required a great deal of my time and energy, and Ana has supported me with every step.

Thank you to my parents, and also to Dragomir and Ljubica Bracilovic, and my uncle Alan for their helpful thoughts and suggestions as they read through the various drafts of this book.

Thank you to my publisher, DiaMedica, and especially its publisher, Dr. Diana M. Schneider. It has been a joy to work with Diana to bring this book to fruition. Her vision and dedication to her work helped to make the entire publishing process smooth and enjoyable. I would also like to thank Jessica Bryan for her outstanding work in editing this book. I am grateful to Richard Lansing for establishing the connection.

*This book is dedicated to my grandparents,
and to the millions of people who have suffered
and who continue to suffer needlessly with arthritis.*

# Preface

I REMEMBER SITTING on the soft, gold rug in my grandma's apartment. It was one of those old rugs that you could run your fingers through, and the threads were always coming loose. But the rug was not so loose or so soft that I couldn't confidently stack my blocks on it in the shape of a small tower that often reached as high as my grandma's knees, as she sat in her favorite armchair. My grandma lived for 92 years, and her life was full and happy—except for the final 20 years of her life, when she was plagued with debilitating knee pain that just kept getting worse.

"Why do you need a cane?" I remember asking her. "It's not a cane—it's really a magic stick," was her reply, always with a twinkle in her eye. But it wasn't the truth. She told a white lie to make me think she wasn't in pain. But she was. I turned to my parents for the truth. "Arthritis" was their one word answer. Grandma had arthritis. But what was "arthritis?" I wasn't sure. I just knew that I didn't like it because it was hurting her.

Years later, I asked why grandma needed a wheelchair. By this time, she was too tired to trick me, or maybe I had gotten too old. "My arthritis just keeps getting worse," she said. "That's what happens when you reach my age."

I vividly recall my grandmother's determination to enjoy life. She smiled every day and laughed as she struggled through her pain. I'm not sure if it was while sitting on her gold rug, wishing

I could make her pain go away, that I first thought about becoming a doctor. Many years later, I often find myself reflecting back on her. What would her life have been like if she had been treated differently for her arthritis? The treatment for her symptoms was pain medication and, later, a cane. She was prescribed a wheelchair when her pain became too disabling for her to walk. At that point, her heart condition kept her from being a candidate for joint replacement surgery. Because my grandmother was treated inadequately for her arthritis, she wasn't able to continue her active lifestyle. How much more would she have been able to enjoy her final years if she had just taken a few simple, relatively easy steps to ease her pain? How many more years might she have lived?

I'll never know the answers to these questions, but I think it is safe to say that, at the very least, she would have been in much less pain, been able to participate in more of the activities she enjoyed, and had an overall better quality of life for her last 20 years. I don't want others to suffer needlessly because they don't have access to reliable information for preventing and treating arthritis. To that sincere aim, I offer this book. I hope you will better understand arthritis after reading it, and follow the recommended steps to treat your symptoms.

Osteoarthritis, and its associated pain, stiffness, and disability, is *not* an inevitable process of aging. It can be (and has been) successfully treated. By following a simple, three-step, manageable plan that incorporates a healthy diet, exercise, and appropriate supplements, you will help yourself avoid the needless suffering that my grandmother and countless others experienced.

Grant Cooper M.D.
New York, New York
2007

# Introduction

CONGRATULATIONS! BY deciding to read this book, you have taken the first step toward freeing yourself from the pain and disability of arthritis.

You probably experience pain and are concerned about your joints. Maybe your knee aches when you sit for too long or walk down a flight of stairs. Perhaps hip pain prevents you from playing a full day of golf. You may have gone to your doctor, who took an X-ray, diagnosed arthritis, and said, "You're getting older. This is normal wear and tear of your joints. It will keep getting worse, and you may eventually need a joint replacement. In the meantime, try taking some ibuprofen or acetaminophen to help ease the pain." Maybe you heard this advice and thought, *"There has to be something more I can do."*

There *is* more you can do. A lot more. If you are like most people, getting back to a pain-free, active lifestyle won't require drugs, injections, or surgery. It will require effort, however, and you'll have to make some lifestyle adjustments. Getting back to a pain-free life will require a combination of common sense advice, an appropriate diet, targeted exercise, and a few carefully selected supplements.

Medicine remains an intricate combination of art and science, but its roots are firmly planted in science. Science lets us "peek under the hood" of the human body. It provides the necessary insight into the anatomy and physiology of the body, and helps us understand how the body breaks down and how different medications interact with our complicated physiology. Science develops injection and surgical approaches; yet, each of us has uniquely different needs and expectations. Each person responds differently to various problems and treatment approaches. This is why medicine remains very much an art.

As an art and science dedicated to treating the human body and relieving it of disease and injury, medicine has become increasingly fragmented. There are literally thousands of medical journals. General practitioners can train to become specialists, specialists can receive even more training to become subspecialists, and subspecialists may have a particular area of interest within their subspecialty. Given this ever-growing field of specialization, you can imagine how increasingly difficult it has become for primary care doctors to keep up.

Although much more is now known about how to treat and prevent arthritis, it has never been more important for you, the patient, to empower yourself. Learn all you can about your condition; have an educated discussion with your doctor; and take the necessary steps to formulate and follow a treatment plan that works for you.

The book is structured as follows:

Part I begins by explaining the nature of arthritis, what joints are, how they function, and how they develop arthritis. By understanding arthritis and how it affects your joints, you will be in the best position to understand what you can do to help repair them. I'll also introduce the four rules of arthritis management. Part I presents a fairly typical case of arthritis and how a doctor might make a diagnosis. If you have already visited your doctor about joint pain, this section should sound familiar. If it doesn't sound familiar, and you had a very different encounter with your doctor, you may want to consider getting another opinion about your joint pain. If you have not seen your doctor yet, this section will give you an idea of what to expect when you do.

Part II introduces the treatment section of the book, beginning with nutrition. You may be surprised to learn that a few dietary modifications can have a big impact on arthritis. In Part II, we'll learn that our mothers were right—*You are what you eat.* What you put in your body really does profoundly impact how it responds to daily challenges and stresses. Part II discusses these dietary modifications in depth, as well as how and why they help relieve the symptoms of arthritis.

Part III explores exercise as a part of arthritis treatment. The importance of an appropriate exercise regimen in getting back to a pain-free, active lifestyle cannot be overemphasized. It may seem counterintuitive to exercise a painful knee. Won't moving the knee just create more pain? Don't worry. Exercising doesn't have to be painful. In Part III, you'll learn how to strengthen your muscles to protect your joints so it won't be painful to participate in the activities you enjoy most, whether it is playing tennis or golf, or chasing after your kids and grandkids.

Part IV reviews the various supplements available to help treat arthritis. A lot of supplement manufacturers make promises that their products will cure your pain. Some people swear by these supplements, but others say they don't work at all. It can be very confusing. I'll sort through it, and tell you which supplements work best, how they work, and why they work. I'll also help you decide if they are right for you.

Finally, in Part V, I'll explain the tools your doctor has at his disposal. My aim is to help you get back to a pain-free, active lifestyle without prescription medication, injections, or surgery—the standard therapies for worsening arthritis—although sometimes they may be necessary. It is helpful to understand the entire spectrum of care—from diet, exercise, and supplements to more invasive options. Appreciating the available treatments will empower you to have an informed, thoughtful discussion with your doctor about all your options.

This book does not replace, and is not meant to replace, professional medical advice. It is important for you to work hand-in-hand with your doctor to arrive at an accurate diagnosis and to formulate a treatment plan that fits *your* needs and expectations. I encourage you to use this book as a basis for talking with your doctor about your joints and the various treatment options available.

Let's start by dispelling the common myth that arthritis is an inevitable part of aging. "Knee pain, back pain, shoulder pain, hip pain…these are all just things that come with age." That's what my grandmother's doctors told her. Maybe you've heard something similar. But, *nothing could be further from the truth*. Don't let anyone, including your doctor, tell you not to worry about your joint pain because it's just "part of getting older." The only things inevitable in life are death and taxes. Arthritis is no more inevitable than heart disease, lung disease, or cancer. It's true that your risk increases with age, but it's not inevitable, and it's certainly a condition that can be treated. Treatment begins with education, and education begins with Part I of this book.

# PART I.

## Getting To Know Your Joints and How Osteoarthritis Develops

BEFORE DISCUSSING the causes, prevention, and treatment of osteoarthritis, we need an accurate definition. The word "arthritis" comes from the Greek word *arthro,* meaning "joint" and *itis,* meaning "inflammation." Thus, it would seem that arthritis is a set of conditions in which a joint is inflamed. However, as tends to happen with broad medical terms, the word has been used and misused in so many ways that it is now used to refer to just about any joint problem (particularly a chronic one) in which inflammation, pain, and/or stiffness is involved.

There are over 120 different kinds of arthritis, the most common of which is *osteoarthritis.* When most people think of the arthritis that comes with increasing age, they are thinking of osteoarthritis. All references in this book to "arthritis" refer to "osteoarthritis," which accounts for more cases than all the other types combined. The U.S. Centers for Disease Control estimates that one in five adults will experience the symptoms of osteoarthritis by the year 2020.

*Osteo* comes from the Greek word *osteon,* meaning bone. Thus, "osteoarthritis" literally means "arthritis of the bone." The main underlying cause of osteoarthritis is degeneration of the cartilage between the joints. We'll talk much more about this later in the book. For now, let's agree that "osteoarthritis" is a term used to describe a joint problem involving the bones of the joint, and that it may include pain, stiffness, and inflammation. With this in mind, we'll begin the first chapter with a discussion of joints.

# Understanding Your Joints

THE JOINTS of the human body truly are remarkable. Without them, we could not sit, stand, run or jump, play Chopin's "Minute Waltz," throw or catch a winning touchdown pass, shake hands, dance the tango, type on a keyboard, or raft down the Colorado River. Each joint in the body delicately balances stability and flexibility, depending on its function. This same delicate balance is also why we suffer when our joints develop a disease such as arthritis and become painful or stiff.

A joint is a location at which two bones make contact and move in relationship to each other; this is called an *articulation*. Most people have 206 bones and 143 joints. Having so many joints provides a lot of flexibility, but each joint is also a potential site of problems such as pain, stiffness, and inflammation. Depending on the joint, it may be fixed, slightly flexible, or more flexible. The skull, for example, is made up of several bones that are joined together by *fixed* joints. The sacroiliac joints that connect our spine to our hips are *slightly flexible*. Other slightly flexible joints include the joints between the vertebrae in our spine. By contrast, our hips, shoulders, knees, and finger joints are examples of *flexible* joints. As a general rule, the more flexible a joint is, and the more weight-bearing responsibility that it has (think of the hip or knee), the more likely that particular joint is to develop arthritis.

There are many different types of flexible joints. For example, the shoulder and hip joints are examples of *ball-and-socket joints*, the most flexible type of joint in the body. If your shoulder weren't so flexible, you would find it very hard to position your hand where you wanted to in space. The price for this flexibility is that these joints are more likely to dislocate than those that are less flexible.

The knee and elbow are examples of *hinge joints,* which function in a way similar to the opening and closing of a car door. The thumbs have *saddle joints* that allow you to pick things up. Your ankles and wrists have *gliding joints* that allow the bones to glide smoothly over each other. The *pivot joints* in your neck allow for side-to-side movement—you can thank your pivot joints for your ability to give a disapproving headshake whenever you want to!

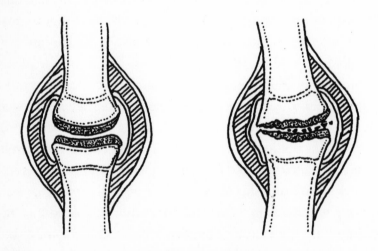

**FIG. 1.1** A NORMAL VS. OSTEOARTHRITIC JOINT.
*Reprinted with permission from The Arthritis Cure, by Theodosakis and Buff, 2003.*

Each mobile joint in your body has the same basic structure (Figure 1.1). The *joint capsule* is on the outside; it is made of tough fibrous tissue that adds strength and stability to the joint and connects the *articulating* bones. A sheet of *synovium* lines the capsule; its cells secrete *synovial fluid*. This fluid, along with water, is the chief constituent of the fluid within the joint. Synovial fluid is thick, straw-colored, and found in small amounts in the joint. The thickness is due in large part to an important component called *hyaluronic acid*. Keep these two words in mind, because injecting hyaluronic acid into the knees and other joints (such as the hips and shoulders) can alleviate symptoms in some people with arthritis. Another important substance inside the joint is called *cartilage*.

## Cartilage

Joints need cartilage to function properly. Up to eight times more slippery than ice, and with the ability to soak up and push out water as easily as a sponge, cartilage is perfectly designed to permit seamless motion between bones, while at the same time providing ideal shock-absorbing capacity. In the world of joints, cartilage is a true superhero. Scientists have put men on the moon, eradicated polio, made flying an everyday event, and decoded DNA, but they haven't yet been able to create a substance that is better suited for joints than the body's own healthy cartilage.

Cartilage is made of *collagen, proteoglycans* (core proteins that are attached to carbohydrate chains), *chondrocytes* (cells that make cartilage), and up to 80 percent water. When you are at rest and your joints are not bearing weight, cartilage stores synovial fluid and water within it. When a joint is loaded with a force, the fluid stored in the cartilage is redistributed to the joint. In other words, when you stand from a seated position, the weight you put on your knee pushes the synovial fluid and water out of the cartilage in your knee, much as it would push the water out of a wet sponge inside your knee. The fluid pushed into the joint space helps to cushion your weight and also nourishes the joint. It moves back into the cartilage when you sit down.

In addition to this sponge-like property, cartilage has another cushioning advantage—it is filled with negatively charged chondroitin molecules. Negative particles resist touching each other with astounding atomic force. When the joint is made to bear weight, these chondroitin molecules are pushed together, but their negative charges resist. Pushing two negatively charged chondroitin molecules together is like trying to force two negatively charged magnets together. The closer they come to touching, the stronger they repel each other.

In osteoarthritis, cartilage degenerates, losing its cushioning and smooth, lubricating effects. As the amount of cartilage decreases, increasing stress is placed on other structures within the joint, such as the bones, joint capsule, ligaments, and tendons.

## MOBILE JOINT ANATOMY—A BRIEF REVIEW

- A tough, fibrous joint capsule on the outside of the joint connects the bones.
- Synovium lines the joint capsule and secretes synovial fluid.
- Synovial fluid lubricates the joint and nourishes the cartilage.
- Cartilage allows for seamless motion between bones and provides shock-absorption.

## THE SUPPORTING STRUCTURES OF BONE

Joints don't work in a vacuum. In order to function properly, they require muscles, tendons, ligaments, and bursae. Let's explore the different parts of the body that interact intimately with the joints:

- ▸ *Muscles* provide the force needed to torque, flex, and extend joints.
- ▸ *Tendons* are tough bands of tissue that attach muscles to bones.
- ▸ *Ligaments* are tough, fibrous bands of tissue that attach bone to bone. In addition to tendons, ligaments cross the joints and help provide stability.
- ▸ *Bursae* are small, fluid-filled sacs that are strategically scattered throughout the body—there are about 160 of them. They contain the same synovial fluid as in joints; they provide cushioning over the bones, ligaments, and muscles. The bursae provide this cushioning in much the same way as bubble wrap provides protection for packages.

When joints are working well, they are one of life's many marvels. All the components of the joint and its supporting structures—bones, ligaments, muscles, tendons, cartilage, bursae, and synovial fluid—work in unison to bring about the intricate movements of a ballerina performing a pirouette as well as the more mundane yet critical functions we all do, including brushing our teeth. However, like many brilliant facts of life, we often take the proper functioning of our joints for granted. We use and abuse them, and only seem to notice them at all when they hurt or become stiff.

Our joints are so important that, when they become diseased and start to lose their normal function, they affect our lives in a profoundly negative way. Any component in a joint can malfunction and cause pain and stiffness. The real problem is that once one part of the joint starts to break down, others tend to follow until a vicious cycle develops. For example, if a ligament is injured, the surrounding muscles have to compensate for the injury. The muscle opposite the injured ligament may have to contract more strongly to take pressure off of the injured side. This increased exertion by the muscle may pull one of the bones slightly to the side, forcing the edges of the two bones to scrape together. This scraping causes inflammation that spreads to the synovium, and so forth. This cycle of destruction leads us to the first two rules of arthritis management:

**Rule #1:** The sooner arthritis is diagnosed and treatment is started, the better.

**Rule #2:** Once symptoms begin, the entire joint, including the surrounding structures, must be treated, including but not limited to the underlying injury.

## CONSIDER RULE #1

Arthritis is a progressive condition when left untreated. If treatment is begun early in the process, you can avoid further degeneration and the need for more aggressive treatments such as drugs and surgery.

## CONSIDER RULE #2

You've had arthritis in your knee for years, but only recently did it start giving you real trouble. During the past few weeks, your knee hurt whenever you climbed even a few stairs or sat for too long. You went to your doctor, who told you what you already knew: your arthritis is acting up. The treatment consists of a steroid injection into your knee.

A steroid is a potent anti-inflammatory medication, and a steroid injection is similar to turning a fire hose on full blast to put out a small fire. The fire goes out, and you feel much better over the next few days and weeks. However, if you don't also address the underlying cause of your arthritis, the symptoms will return. In addition, when the symptoms recur, the underlying damage to the joint will have progressed, and the pain may be worse than before. Because the arthritis has progressed, a steroid injection may not work as well the second or third time. Thus, the entire joint and its surrounding structures must be treated so the symptoms will go away and stay away.

## THE SYNOVIAL FLUID

Synovial fluid is necessary for normal joint function. As discussed previously, synovial fluid moves into the cartilage when a joint is resting, and moves out into the joint space when the joint is active, particularly when the joint is engaged in a weight-bearing activity such as exercise. Synovial fluid lubricates the joints and permits smooth movement. It also provides important nutrients to them.

Joints are not *vascularized,* meaning that they have no direct blood supply. They get banged around a lot; bleeding could occur inside a joint every time it was injured if blood flowed through it. Even if blood had a quick escape route from the joints (which it does not), tough, fibrous scar tissue would develop and impair future functioning. Instead, the joint capsule receives limited blood by diffusion, which allows nutrients and waste products to be exchanged within the synovial fluid inside the joint.

If we don't use our joints, however, the synovial fluid remains within the cartilage and cannot interact with the joint capsule. Until the joints are stressed with movement and weight, their needs will be not be met. This brings us to the third rule of arthritis management:

**Rule #3:** Joints require movement to maintain optimal health and function.

---

## THE BENEFITS OF THE THIRD RULE

Following the third rule of arthritis management will help ensure that the joint receives adequate nutrients and that waste products will be removed. It will also help ensure that the muscles and other supporting structures around the joint are exercised and strengthened. When muscles around a joint are strong, they take some of the pressure off the joint. When muscles are weak, the static joint must bear the increased pressure.

---

Having agreed that arthritis is a joint problem that may include pain, stiffness, and inflammation, having discussed what a joint is, and having introduced the first three rules of arthritis management, we are now ready to discuss how arthritis develops.

# How Joints Develop Arthritis

CARTILAGE DEGENERATION is the primary underlying problem in arthritis. As discussed in Chapter 1, the smoothness of the cartilage allows for easy gliding between joints. Its sponginess allows synovial fluid and water to enter it during times of rest and rapidly exit when the joint is stressed by walking or other activity. The movement of these fluids provides the shock-absorbing capacity of the joint as well as the nourishment it needs.

There are two basic types of osteoarthritis: primary and secondary.

## SECONDARY ARTHRITIS

In secondary arthritis, something identifiable triggers the degradation of the cartilage. In other words, the arthritis *follows* the injury. This type of arthritis is seen in people who have suffered a severe trauma or repetitive microtrauma to a joint. They may be obese or overexert themselves (such as running a marathon without proper training). They may have abnormal *body biomechanics*, a term that refers to how the skeletal structures, including the bones, muscles, tendons, ligaments, and joints, function together—meaning how they move through space under the influence of gravity.

People with a history of severe joint trauma, such as a broken bone or a torn knee ligament, may have suffered cartilage damage at the time of injury. This damage initiates a process of degeneration that can cause further cartilage damage and erosion. People who suffer repetitive microtrauma, such as a runner who wears improper footwear, may experience continual microtrauma to the joint cartilage.

Once cartilage in the joint has been damaged, the cells that make the cartilage (chondrocytes) fill the small or large cracks created by trauma with new cartilage. Unfortunately, this new tissue is inferior to normal cartilage, and it is more likely to crack and overgrow into places where it's not needed, interfering with normal functioning. This sets the stage for further abnormal joint biomechanics.

Whenever the biomechanics of a joint are abnormal, increased stress is placed on parts of the joint that are not designed to deal with it, including bones, ligaments, and the joint capsule. More bone is added in response to these stresses for protection and cushioning. Bone is far from inanimate or static; quite the contrary, it is very much alive and dynamic. Bones are constantly breaking down and being rebuilt. When they are forced to take on the shock-absorbing role of cartilage, they create new bone in an effort to strengthen the joint. These extra pieces of bone are called *bone spurs*. They can rub against the surrounding muscles, tendons, ligaments, and synovium, causing irritation and inflammation. As the joint becomes inflamed and painful, you are more likely to avoid using it, leading to greater stiffness, a loss of critical nutrients, and atrophy of the surrounding muscles.

The muscles that surround joints are responsible for taking some of the load off them, particularly the weight-bearing joints. Atrophy and weakness of these muscles means they can no longer buffer the joint, which then has to carry an increased load. This leads to further breakdown, which leads to further pain, which leads to further disuse and more atrophy. Thankfully, strengthening the surrounding muscles can have a profound impact in taking the extra load off the joints, thereby reducing the downward spiral.

Obesity and overexertion can cause repetitive trauma to the cartilage. In overexertion, the surrounding muscles become fatigued, and the joints are forced to face increased loads. Joints are designed to accommodate temporary increases in load but—despite their elegant design, they do have limits. Lifting too much weight while squatting, jumping onto a very hard surface, or other sudden increases in load on a joint can lead to cartilage injury. As with other injuries, once the cartilage is damaged, it is more likely to suffer subsequent damage.

## Body Biomechanics

When the body functions optimally, weight is distributed so that weak structures bear less weight and stronger structures bear more. The biomechanics of the body are incredibly complex and, at the same time, sublimely simple. They are complex because of all the factors involved: the movement of the joints—the muscles pushing and pulling, the ligaments stretching and straining, and all the different angles and forces. They are simple because the body is designed to function logically and smoothly.

Understanding the core concept of body biomechanics is to understand that all the parts of the body are connected, and that a force directed at one part affects the rest. When you take a step, the impact of the force on your heel as it strikes the ground is transmitted up your leg to your knee. If your knee does not cushion and absorb the force, it will be redistributed to your hip. If your hip does not cushion and absorb the force, it will travel across your pelvis, and so forth.

Most people do not move with perfect body biomechanics. For example, most of us lift objects in a way that is not optimal from a biomechanical perspective: we bend over and lift from the hips and lower back, instead of keeping the back straight and bending from the knees. Only when we start to feel pain in the lower back and talk to a friend or a doctor about it, do we learn how to bend properly to take the load off the lower back and redistribute it where it belongs: in the lower limbs and muscles. Even once we've learned this important, pain-saving body biomechanical skill, most people revert to their old ways once the pain is gone…only to be injured again. Eventually, they either adopt the new biomechanics or stop lifting heavy objects.

Poor body biomechanics can be inherited or acquired, rather than learned. For example, if you have a flat foot, you will not have the benefit of a proper foot arch to redistribute your body weight when you walk and climb stairs. Instead of the weight being dissipated in part by the arch of the foot, the load is dispersed inappropriately to the foot, knee, and hip. This occurs because your biomechanics have been altered to the point that structures not designed to consistently accept greater loads are forced to do so. Fortunately, while a higher arch can't be "learned," an arch support inside the shoe to redistribute the weight properly can help restore proper biomechanics. Often, this is all that is needed to relieve the pain.

There are countless ways in which body biomechanics can be disrupted. One of the more common reasons is tight, contracted, and/or weak muscles. The forces generated by muscles take weight off the joints and keep them aligned. Weak muscles can't adequately support a joint, which allows the joint to slip and slide under the force of the body's weight. In this case, the weight may come to rest on the weaker, more static parts of the joint instead of the stronger ones that are designed to take the brunt of the load.

A tight or contracted muscle cannot adequately protect the joint from the stresses of daily life, and it can also cause damage by exerting a constant force on the joint, pulling it out of alignment and forcing parts of the joint to bear weight it wasn't meant to take. The tight muscle also changes your body posture, placing increasing loads on multiple joints. For example, if your hip flexors are tight (which is very common) your pelvis and spine are constantly being pulled forward, increasing stress. When the pelvis and spine are pulled forward, the muscles attaching to the back of them (particularly the lower back muscles) are stretched and forced to work much harder to pull the spine back into alignment. Because the hip flexors are the strongest muscles in the body, the lower back muscles eventually fatigue, stretch, and may become inflamed. While this tug of war is going on between your muscles, tendons, and ligaments, the joints of your pelvis and spine are out of proper position. Their individual components, which include the sacro-iliac joint, discs of the spine, and small posterior facet joints of the spine, also are pulled out of position and forced to redistribute the load of the body weight in a suboptimal manner.

Once proper body biomechanics are disrupted, for whatever reason, it is important to restore them as much as possible. Simple things such as finding the right foot orthotic, stretching the hip flexors and other muscles, strengthening weak muscles, learning to bend properly, and correcting posture, can make an enormous difference in slowing the progression of arthritis, reducing pain, and improving quality of life. This will be discussed in more depth in the section about exercises that can help prevent and treat arthritis.

## PRIMARY ARTHRITIS

The causes of primary arthritis are not as well understood. In contrast to secondary arthritis, primary arthritis occurs without any directly identifiable cause. Primary arthritis tends to occur after the age of 45, and it becomes more common with advancing age. Arthritis tends to run in families, and most experts believe that it may have a genetic component. It seems reasonable that primary arthritis results from some combination of repetitive microtrauma to the joint, impaired or suboptimal biomechanics, and other un-identified factors, such as a potential genetic predisposition or environmental factors.

## Cartilage Degeneration

As mentioned previously, cartilage does not have a direct blood supply. It also does not have a nerve supply. Nerves transmit information within the body, and without them you would not know where your body is in space (*proprioceptive* nerves), or when your body is in pain or has been injured (*nociceptive* nerves). Pain alerts us to the fact that the body needs attention. However, many parts of the body do not have nerve endings. The brain, for example, has little need to transmit pain signals because it is protected by the bones of the cranium.

If cartilage had nerve endings, the daily pushing, pulling, and twisting that occurs within normal, healthy joints would result in pain, making movement difficult. Furthermore, arthritis is less of a significant issue from an evolutionary standpoint because most people don't develop this condition until they are over the age of 55—although hard labor and injuries can predispose a person to early secondary arthritis. Until recently, most people didn't live this long. Now that we live longer, healthier, and more active lives, arthritis has become a more significant and distressing disease.

Although cartilage doesn't have nerve endings, bone, synovium, the joint capsule, and the surrounding muscles, tendons, and ligaments do. As cartilage becomes severely worn, pressure and stress accumulate in the surrounding structures, creating friction and inflammation. As it degenerates and inferior cartilage is created, water gradually fills the void. This increased aqueous presence in the joint does not have the same shock-absorbing or sponge-like properties, or the icy smoothness of cartilage. As the cartilage becomes further damaged, the ligaments, joint capsule, tendons, muscles, and bones are forced to bear undue weight, and the nerve endings in these structures begin to transmit pain.

## OSTEOARTHRITIS: THE SILENT KILLER OF JOINTS

Doctors often call high blood pressure the "silent killer," because you don't typically feel high blood pressure. For this reason, it is critically important that doctors screen their patients for high blood pressure and treat it appropriately to avoid a stroke or heart attack.

If high blood pressure is the silent killer of hearts and brains, arthritis can be thought of as the "silent killer" of joints, because cartilage degeneration in and of itself is painless.

## INFLAMMATION

We have all experienced inflammation at one time or other. You stub your toe and it gets red, hot, and swollen. You twist your ankle and the next day it is swollen and painful. What causes these symptoms?

The word *inflammation* comes from the Latin word "inflammatio," meaning to set on fire. Inflammation is a complex, biological response by the body to harmful stimuli, including bacteria, viruses, fungus, irritants, and physical injury. It is the body's way of protecting us and promoting healing. Symptoms of inflammation in a joint include swelling, redness, pain when the joint is touched, stiffness, and loss of function.

Some types of arthritis are *autoimmune* diseases, such as rheumatoid arthritis, shoulder tendonitis or bursitis, gouty arthritis, and polymyalgia rheumatica. In these diseases, inflammation is caused by an inappropriate response by the immune system in which the white blood cells attack joint tissue.

Inflammation in the synovial membrane occurs in osteoarthritis, and results in the production of tissue-damaging free radicals.

## Free Radicals and Antioxidants

Free radicals are produced when weak molecular bonds are attacked and broken, resulting in a molecule with an unpaired electron. This unpaired electron is extremely unstable and quickly "attacks" a neighboring molecule to capture its electron, resulting in the next compound losing its electron, and so on. This sets up a rapid cycle that can quickly cascade into the destruction of the living cell. This process is called the *oxidative response*, and the resulting free radicals are capable of producing extensive tissue damage. Fortunately, substances called *antioxidants* can slow or prevent the oxidation of other chemicals and prevent damage to the cells. Plants and animals maintain complex systems of different types of antioxidants, including vitamins C and E. The importance of eating foods high in natural antioxidants and taking supplements when necessary is discussed in Part II.

## Subchondral Cysts

In addition to inflammation, damage to the bones is ongoing in osteoarthritis. In essence, sensing the increasing pressure and inflammation, the bones harden (sclerose) and enlarge their defensive perimeter of bone tissue. As the bones enlarge and become sclerotic, fluid-filled pockets can form beneath them. These pockets are called *subchondral cysts*. The new hard surface created by the bone becomes a further source of irritation, rubbing and scratching the structures around it and perpetuating the cycle of inflammation and damage.

This cycle doesn't have to become self-perpetuating—it *can* be broken. This brings us back to the first rule of arthritis management: The sooner arthritis is diagnosed and treatment is started, the better.

# 3.

## Obesity and Arthritis

PEOPLE WHO are obese have a significantly increased risk of developing arthritis, because obesity is an important source of chronic microtrauma to the cartilage. Joints are designed for carrying, properly distributing, and cushioning body weight. They are also capable of taking on temporary excess loads. For example, stress on the joints is greatly increased when we carry groceries, lift weights, bend over, or run up stairs. However, joints do have limits.

Each step you take while walking involves temporarily transferring your weight primarily onto one joint. When you factor in momentum, biomechanics, and gravity, your knees and hips experience up to three times as much pressure as your body weight with each step. If you weigh 140 pounds, your knee joints may experience as much as 320 pounds of weight with each step. When you walk down a flight of stairs, your hip and knee joints may experience as much as a six-fold increase in weight, so that same 140-pound person experiences as much as 640 pounds across the knees and hips.

In other words, every pound you gain punishes your joints up to six-fold. Research clearly bears this out; overweight men are five times more likely to develop arthritis, and overweight women are four times more likely to develop it than are their non-overweight counterparts. For every 10 pounds of excess weight gain, the risk of developing arthritis increases by 40 percent.

Every time you take a step, the extra weight places increased pressure on your weight-bearing joints, because the load is too great for your muscles, ligaments, and tendons. The joints shift under the weight and, ultimately, they are overwhelmed, resulting in repetitive microtears in the cartilage. Additional stresses are taken up by static portions of your bone, creating friction. Your bone responds by trying to build new bone, but the new bone is weaker than the original bone, and the process of arthritis is well on its way.

## HORMONES MAY BE A FACTOR

In addition to the mechanical forces created by obesity, it may also contribute to arthritis through hormonal influences that are not yet clearly understood. Studies have found a strong link between obesity and arthritis of the hip and knee, with a weaker link between obesity and arthritis of the hand. Since the hand does not experience significantly increased mechanical pressures in obesity, and because it is not a significant weight-bearing joint, other factors may also be at work, such as hormonal differences. Estrogen levels are increased in obesity, in addition to other hormonal imbalances.

## THE CYCLE OF PAIN AND WEIGHT GAIN

You may be less inclined to exercise as joint pain increases. This decreased activity in turn leads to further weight gain, which leads to increased stress on the joints, causing more pain, less movement, and more weight gain. This is a difficult cycle to break. Fortunately, there is hope. Once you start shedding excess weight, you will take a significant amount of stress off your joints, and this will lead to a significant decrease in pain and stiffness.

If you are obese and worried about the damage you may have already done to your joints, lose weight now and you will greatly reduce your chances of developing arthritis. Women who lose as little as 11 pounds reduce their risk of developing arthritis of the knee by more than 50 percent.

The good news is that many of the same steps to treat and prevent arthritis will also help you shed excess weight with no extra effort. If you're obese or overweight, you already know that you should lose weight, and a doctor has probably already told you that it is important for you to lose weight. You may have tried different diets and found it difficult to shed the pounds. Please don't despair. Once you start eating right and exercising, as described in the treatment sections of this book, the weight will start to come off. You'll be amazed by how much better your joints will feel.

# 4

# Making the Diagnosis

I F YOU have joint pain, you should see your doctor to find out why. Only your doctor can give you an accurate diagnosis, and thus prevent you from receiving the wrong treatment. Many problems besides osteoarthritis can cause joint pain and/or stiffness, including other types of arthritis, infection, bone disease, cancer, fracture, and injury to the ligaments. Treatment is specific for each disease and for each individual. Your doctor can look at your medical history, perform a comprehensive physical examination, and order the necessary tests.

With this in mind, let's consider a typical case of arthritis. The patient described below is really a composite of several different people. We'll discuss her symptoms, which may sound familiar, and how she would typically be evaluated.

## JANET'S STORY

Janet was a 67-year-old mother of four and grandmother of two. She visited my office complaining of right knee pain. "It started about a year ago," she said, shaking her head and looking down at her knee. "At first, I thought it was just one of those aches that comes with getting older. It would hurt at the end of the day but then it would get better. For a while, it seemed to go away. But then it would come back. I would rub it and the pain would go away slowly. Then the pain started coming in the middle of the day, or whenever I went up and down stairs. Stairs were the worst. It got to the point where I didn't want to do anything. Now the pain lasts for hours, and sometimes it's even hard to fall asleep. What really upsets me is that I can't play with my grandchildren. They're 6 and 7 years old now. I used to get on the floor and play with them. I haven't been able to do that for over a year. It's just terrible."

Janet's story is classic for arthritis of the knee, so I asked her why it had taken her so long to see a doctor.

"I went to see my primary care doctor months ago," she said. "He took some X-rays and told me I had arthritis but that it wasn't too advanced yet. He said arthritis was part of getting older but that, if it got bad enough, I could talk to a surgeon about replacing my whole knee. Her doctor told my friend Alice the same thing. I don't want to have surgery. My doctor told me to take an over-the-counter painkiller, but it doesn't help enough and I'm in a lot of pain."

Janet's situation is common. People go to their doctor for help with pain and are told there is not much that can be done besides taking over-the-counter medications. If the pain gets bad enough, they're told surgery is the next option. Arthritis is *not* inevitable. The more aggressive we are in preventing and treating the early symptoms, the more we can reduce the probability of developing arthritis and/or allowing it to worsen.

The second point of importance from Janet's story is that the degree of severity of disease on an X-ray often does not correlate with symptoms. A person with a terrible looking X-ray of the knee may be completely symptom-free. Likewise, a person who shows minimal arthritis on an X-ray may be experiencing severe pain. This does not mean that one person is stoic and the other is a complainer. Different people have higher or lower thresholds for pain, depending on their body biochemistry and the synapses within their brain. Many factors influence the pain threshold in a given individual, including social support, depression, painful stimuli, and other potential biochemical and neuromodulating factors.

Someone who has severe cartilage degeneration may not have reached the point where the surrounding structures have become irritated and inflamed. As discussed previously, if only cartilage is involved, there will be no pain because cartilage doesn't have any nerve endings. By contrast, the person with minimal X-ray findings of cartilage degeneration may just be unlucky enough to have the cartilage degrade in a pattern that allows pressure to be placed on the surrounding structures, leading to irritation and inflammation. Perhaps the synovium was already inflamed, or perhaps the bone was already compensating for increased pressure, and a tiny bone spur hooked a piece of the joint capsule or irritated a ligament. Whenever I am teaching a medical student or junior doctor, I always emphasize the fourth rule of arthritis management:

**Rule #4:** Make sure you treat the patient, not the X-ray.

In essence, the presence of asymptomatic findings of arthritis on an X-ray should be taken as a warning that the joint is not healthy and will probably become painful if you don't start taking better care of it. This is analogous to getting a routine electrocardiogram (EKG) to look at your heart before a surgery for your stomach and finding slight heart damage. While anyone can develop heart disease, and everyone should take good care of his heart, the presence of heart damage on an EKG should prompt you to start taking better care of your heart immediately.

Always treat the patient, not the X-ray. A person with no clinical symptoms and X-ray findings of arthritis should be treated in the same way as someone with no symptoms and no X-ray findings. Both should eat right, exercise, and take the appropriate supplements. The key difference is that the person with X-ray findings may be at greater risk of developing symptoms sooner, and should take preventative measures as soon as possible. Routine screening with X-rays to look for arthritis damage is definitely not indicated because they expose the patient to unnecessary radiation and are costly.

## X-ray Findings of Arthritis in the Absence of Symptoms

Sometimes, X-rays are taken for other reasons besides joint pain, and arthritis is incidentally seen on the film. Joint pain may be present, but a cause of the pain other than arthritis is ultimately identified. Noticing signs of arthritis on X-ray should nevertheless prompt a greater sense of urgency for the patient to take steps to reduce the risk of developing worsening arthritis, which likely will eventually lead to pain and suffering if it is not appropriately managed.

Janet's future is much brighter than she suspects. It would have been better if she had seen a specialist in the treatment of arthritis or sports medicine earlier. However, many effective yet conservative nonsurgical treatments are available to help her.

In order to properly diagnose Janet, I would have asked more questions. I would want to know if any of her other joints hurt, and whether she was experiencing any other pain or symptoms. Night sweats, flushing, fever, chills, history of a fall that precipitated the pain, recent unintended weight loss, pain that wakes her up at night, pain in both knees that started at the same time, and multiple joint pains are just some of the symptoms that would make me concerned about another underlying disease process. For example, night sweats, fevers, and chills would suggest that Janet might have an infection or other systemic illness. (*Systemic* means the entire body is affected.) Pain that wakes her from sleeping and/or recent unintended weight loss might suggest cancer.

As with any patient, I would take a complete medical history. This would include asking her about other medical conditions and what prescription and over-the-counter medications she takes, including supplements. I would also ask questions about whether she has any allergies, her home environment, and her relationships.

## Physical Examination

Next, I would perform a thorough physical examination. I would start by watching how Janet walks. How is her posture and alignment? Are her feet turned in or out; does she have flat feet or too high an arch? Does she bend or lean to one side? I would perform a comprehensive musculoskeletal and neurologic examination. I would want to know, in particular, whether she has any weakness or tightness, and I would want to make sure she has no neurologic problems.

Certain findings during my examination might lead me toward another diagnosis. For example, joint tenderness in her knee would lead me to consider a meniscus tear, which might prompt me to order magnetic resonance imaging (MRI). Warmth and a significant amount of swelling in the joint would suggest a possible infection. If rotating her hip reproduced her knee pain, I would suspect the true pathology might be in her hip, not her knee. These are just a few of the many considerations addressed during a thorough physical examination.

Finally, I would be sure to examine Janet's shoes. As mentioned previously, footwear is often the culprit in causing or contributing to pain.

If Janet's history and physical examination confirmed the diagnosis of arthritis, I would order X-rays of her knee. These X-rays would be more to confirm my diagnosis than to arrive at a diagnosis, and they would help establish the extent of cartilage degeneration. MRI would actually be a better tool to evaluate the integrity of the cartilage, because it can look at the soft tissues of the body. However, MRI is an expensive, time-intensive test that her insurance would probably not cover for this purpose. Furthermore, the MRI findings would not change my management recommendations; they would only be for future use to mark the progression of the arthritis.

In practice, X-rays are more than sufficient for the task at hand. They can show bone spurs (osteophytes), subchondral cysts (the fluid-filled cysts that sometimes occur beneath the hardened bone), and joint space narrowing (the most classic finding in arthritis of the knee). As the cartilage degenerates, the bones move closer and closer together until they actually grind into each other. X-rays can mark this progression, although hopefully measures will be taken to slow or halt the progression once it is identified.

As emphasized earlier, X-rays may not correlate with the degree of symptoms. A treatment plan should be based on the severity of the symptoms, not X-ray findings. X-rays allow doctors to follow the progression or remission of disease and give an idea as to the extent of the anatomic damage that has already occurred.

## DIAGNOSTIC TESTING

X-rays and computed tomography (CT) scans are primarily used to visualize bony structures. CT scans actually use multiple specialized X-rays to view the body area from different angles and then give multiple cross-sectional images of it. The benefits of better visualization offered by CT over X-ray must be weighed against the risks of significantly increased radiation exposure and increased time and costs of the procedure.

Neither CT nor X-ray is as good at looking at soft tissues (cartilage, nerves, and organs) as MRI scans. MRI does not use radiation, but rather radio waves and magnetic fields. The major drawbacks of routine MRI usage are the time and expense of the procedure. It may be uncomfortable for some people because it can produce claustrophobia.

X-rays and CT scans should be avoided in women who are pregnant or planning to become pregnant. Women who are pregnant should talk to their doctor before having an MRI; at the time of this writing, there is no clear risk of MRI for pregnancy, but many doctors as well as many patients prefer to play it safe and not use MRI until after pregnancy.

There are other contraindications to X-ray, CT, and MRI, as well as other imaging modalities (PET and ultrasound). For example, a patient with metal in his body cannot have an MRI. Discuss all the risks and benefits of any test with your doctor to find out if it's right for you.

Now that arthritis has been defined and you understand how it develops and how it appears clinically, you are ready for Part II, which focuses on the first part of any good treatment plan: nutrition.

# Nutrition

NUTRITION HAS a profound impact on the entire body, including the joints. This section will teach you how to follow a "joint-healthy" diet. The same good nutritional habits that will help repair your joints will also help keep your heart healthy, reduce your risk of cancer and other diseases, give you more energy, and improve your outlook on life. Can changing your diet really do all that? You bet your joints it can!

You may be struck by how much of what I say sounds like common sense. That's because it *is*. If you think you've heard some of this before, you probably have. I'll explain the evidence behind a joint-healthy diet as well as how eating right helps your joints. We will also discuss less well-known information, such as why having more boron in your diet may reduce your risk of arthritis. Let's start our discussion about nutrition with a lesson from abroad.

## A HEALTHY DIET EMPHASIZES FRESH FOODS

My wife's family is from Yugoslavia. Growing up in New Jersey, she often returned with her parents and brother to visit her extended family there. During the summer, she enjoyed eating the many varieties of local fruits and vegetables. Throughout the rest of the year, her house would be filled by her mother with fresh meats, cheeses, fruits, and vegetables from local farmers markets, always prepared with great attention to detail. Whenever I visited her parents' home, there was always a wonderfully rich smell of home-cooked food in the air. My mother-in-law describes one major difference between eating in America and how she used to eat while growing up in Yugoslavia:

"When I was a girl, we didn't go to the market knowing what we wanted to buy. My mother went to the market to see what was fresh, and *that* was what she bought. Here, we go to the supermarket and get whatever we want, because we have foods from all over the world. But," she shakes her head, "I don't think it's always so fresh."

I also grew up in New Jersey. My parents were "health-conscious," but being health-conscious then was very different from what it is now, because we didn't have the same level of information. We always had a home-cooked dinner (except Fridays, which was often pizza night). Like most of my friends, my lunch consisted of peanut butter and jelly sandwiches on white bread. Usually, there would also be a tasty, colorful snack with too much sugar.

The first time I experienced culture shock was when I met my wife in high school:

"What do you mean you never had white bread?" I asked her, genuinely confused.

"I didn't know anyone ate that stuff," was her sincere reply. "It's so artificial."

## A Return to Basics

A lot can be learned from this food culture clash. Europeans in general have very different eating habits from Americans. Different doesn't always mean better, but consider the fact that America's obesity rate is higher than almost any other country. Despite spending twice as much per person on healthcare, and the superior medical technology at our disposal, Americans suffer as many or more heart attacks and other diseases as Europeans. It seems reasonable, therefore, to return to basics in order to discover what we might be missing.

It doesn't get much more basic than diet. When we look at the average American diet, it immediately becomes apparent—both from a common sense perspective as well as a researched medical one—that we have a lot to learn from our neighbors across the Atlantic about what we should and should not be putting into our bodies.

The chapters in this section offer dietary guidelines for improving health and alleviating the symptoms of arthritis.

# 5.

## Nutrition Overview—
## Getting Started with the Cure

L ET'S COVER a few basic principles before discussing the specific foods that contribute to a generally healthful and, more specifically, a joint-healthy, anti-inflammatory diet. If you do nothing else but follow these basic principles, you will be healthier and your symptoms will probably improve.

### THE FIVE NUTRITION BASICS

- Drink plenty of fluids, mostly water.
- Eat more fruits and vegetables.
- Eat more cold-water fish.
- Eat red meat sparingly.
- Eat fewer processed foods.

A note of caution: If you become too concerned about exactly how many milligrams of a specific nutrient there is in the food you eat each day, you are likely to become overwhelmed and discouraged. You will do better if you keep the Five Nutrition Basics in mind. This is not to say that you shouldn't have a detailed understanding of the nutrients you need. On the contrary, knowledge will give you the power to better pick and choose your diet, as well as understand why you should eat specific foods.

Stay true to the basic principles and choose foods that fit your diet and taste good. If you don't enjoy the food you eat, you will always feel as if you are "dieting," instead of just enjoying a healthy diet, which is your ultimate goal. Here is a brief explanation of the Five Nutrition Basics. They will be discussed in more depth in the coming chapters.

## DRINK PLENTY OF FLUIDS, MOSTLY WATER

Fluids are essential to the proper functioning of the body. Body mass is made up of about 60 percent water in men and 55 percent in women (this difference is due to the higher percentage of body fat in women). Blood is over 80 percent water; body fat contains about 25 percent water; and even our brain is about 70 percent water. There is no such thing as being "bone dry," because almost a quarter of bone mass is water. Sufficient water is critical to human health and function.

## EAT MORE FRUITS AND VEGETABLES

Fruits and vegetables are full of the important vitamins and nutrients we need for optimal health and function. Vitamins A, C, and E, selenium, boron, and other nutrients are essential antioxidants that help our bodies fight infection and inflammation.

## EAT MORE COLD-WATER FISH

Cold-water fish contain a high percentage of omega–3 fatty acids, including alpha-linolenic acid, eicosapentaenoic acid (EPA), and docosahexaenoic acid (DHA). Your body contains billions of cells, and every one of them has fatty acids in its outer wall (membrane). Fatty acids are also metabolized into proteins and hormones, and they have a profound effect on the way cells interact with one another. Cells are constantly dying, regenerating, dividing, and changing their shape. The fatty acids that you consume today find their way into your cells and proteins tomorrow. You are, in a very real and immediate sense, what you eat.

Fatty acids are found in many foods—fish, meat, oils, and vegetables. The fatty acids in fish have many potential benefits, including anti-inflammatory effects. Omega-3 fatty acids also appear to improve heart health, because fish oils help to keep platelets from sticking together and forming the plaques in arteries that cause heart disease and peripheral vascular disease. They fight depression, improve insulin sensitivity, and potentially aid in cancer prevention. Research in many of these areas is ongoing. However, some of the strongest evidence supports the anti-inflammatory, anti-arthritis capabilities of a diet high in omega-3 fatty acids. It is important to eat the smaller cold-water fish, such as canned light tuna, salmon, and pollock, because the larger, predatory fish—such as shark, swordfish, and king mackerel, contain a higher percentage of mercury.

## Eat Red Meat Sparingly

The fatty acids in red meat are proinflammatory and damaging to your blood vessels and heart. Therefore, it is best to eat more cold-water fish and less red meat.

## Eat Fewer Processed Foods

Processed foods are, well, processed. As intelligent as we are; as scientifically and technologically advanced as we have become; and as motivated as we are for self-improvement as a species, we have not even come close to matching Mother Nature's ability to nourish us. The foods we create in the laboratory are not as nutritious as those grown on a farm. When hospitalized patients can't swallow and must be given long-term supplementation directly into their stomach or blood, they may develop kidney, liver, metabolic, and gastrointestinal disorders because the nutritional mixture that we are able to manufacture is inadequate. Ultimately, food is the most nutritious when it is carefully looked after, grown, and cultivated, particularly fruits and vegetables. For example, corn, tomatoes, grapes, cucumbers, and just about every other vegetable and fruit we now take for granted, would not exist in its current form without human intervention.

Processed foods typically have more sugar, fat (typically of the bad, omega-6 type), and chemicals than fresh foods, and fewer vitamins and minerals. Many of the chemicals in processed foods may seem to be benign, but they may prove one day to be dangerous. We simply, and perhaps ominously, do not know yet.

Let's take a more detailed look at each of the Five Nutrition Basics.

# 6.

## Drink Plenty of Fluids, Mostly Water

THE SUN was dancing across the flower petals and casting small shadows all around the college students, who were lying on blankets, throwing Frisbees, and doing the typical things that college students do. I was a junior at Princeton University, and I wanted to do only two things on that very pleasant Friday afternoon: study my class notes and relax with my friends. But I could do neither. Like many others on campus at the time, I had come down with what seemed to be the flu. I was feverish, my throat hurt, and I was fatigued. I went to the student health center, hoping they would help me. Perhaps some antibiotics? An injection of some sort?

The nurse practitioner at the clinic knew my symptoms before I had even listed them. Apparently, this "bug" was going around. "It won't respond to antibiotics," she said. "It's a virus and all you can do is to wait it out. You'll feel better in a few days."

*A few days?* I was very disappointed. But she was not without important, and unbeknownst to either of us, life-changing advice. "Drink water," she told me.

I nodded. "I've been drinking water," I said. In truth, at the time I wasn't much of a water drinker at all. Water, to me, often meant whatever existed in a glass of soda, juice, or milk.

"No." The nurse shook her head. "You're dehydrated. When I say drink water, I mean drink A LOT of water." She held up a 1.5 liter bottle. "Drink at least four of these immediately."

I left the clinic feeling dejected. When I got back to my room, I felt so miserable that I decided to take the nurse's advice. *Water couldn't hurt*, I thought. I wasn't feeling thirsty, but I was surprised how easily it went down. Even before I started feeling full, I had drunk two liters, and I began to feel better, so I drank two more liters.

What happened next stunned me. I no longer felt feverish; my throat didn't hurt; and my fatigue lifted like the clearing of a morning fog. I remember shaking my head in disbelief, grabbing a book and another bottle of water, and going outside to join my friends. It was amazing, and it sold me forever on the potential healing powers of water. I started reading about water and dehydration to find out why water is so important to the human body.

## The Restorative Effects of Water

Years later, I often find myself explaining the restorative traits of water to others. Our bodies have amazing antibacterial, antiviral, and antifungal capabilities. A huge array of white blood cells has been specifically designed for our body's defense, including those that fight infection. We can eat healthy food and take as many supplements as we want, but the body needs water to live and function optimally. The importance of good hydration cannot be overestimated.

## How Much Water Does the Body Need?

The American Heart Association recommends drinking 6 to 8 glasses of water per day to maintain the fluid balance of someone who is healthy and relatively inactive. However, people with arthritis often need more. Pure water is best, but sports drinks are also a reasonable choice provided they are the type that replenishes electrolytes, not sugary substitutes. Juices are good sources of water and vitamins, but they have more calories. Sodas, coffee, and other drinks that contain caffeine should be reduced or avoided, because caffeine is a diuretic that can cause you to lose much of the fluid you take in.

Mild to moderate dehydration is extremely common. It seems reasonable to suspect that you would feel thirst before becoming dehydrated, or at least soon after becoming dehydrated. However, thirst is not a good indicator of the body's fluid status. Despite the fact that people can survive for weeks without food, and only a few days without any water, our hunger drive is much greater than our thirst drive. If you wait to feel thirsty, chances are that you are already dehydrated. So drink up and be sure to stay well hydrated.

## Alcohol

Alcohol is also a diuretic, not to mention having a lot of calories if it is part of a mixed drink. If you do drink alcohol, drink it in moderation and consider drinking red wine. Red wine is made with grape skins (white wine is not), and the skin contains polyphenols, which are powerful antioxidants. Drinking red wine in moderation (1–2 glasses per day for men and 1 glass per day for women) decreases blood pressure and may reduce the risk of a heart attack. However, wine is loaded with empty calories.

Alcohol has many negative effects on the body, including raising the level of triglycerides (a risk factor for heart attack and stroke). It also has negative effects on the liver. If you are considering taking a daily glass of wine because of its potential health benefits, check with your physician, because different medications and medical conditions interact with wine in a variety of ways.

# 7

# Eat More Fruits and Vegetables

YOU'VE PROBABLY heard it since you were a child: "An apple a day keeps the doctor away," "Eat carrots because they're good for your eyes," "You can have dessert after you finish your peas…" Guess what? Your parents were right! Eating more fruits and vegetables will help keep you healthy. Since we all know it's the right thing to do, and we all tell each other it's the right thing to do, why do so few of us actually do it?

Could it be that we just don't care about our health? If that were true, you wouldn't be reading this book, and I wouldn't have written it. Maybe we're hoping for a short cut. After all, so many supplements are available. Can't we just take two of them and then go straight to the ice cream aisle? Why eat an orange when you can take a vitamin C pill? Do you have to eat your carrots if you can take a beta-carotene pill?

Yes, you do, because whole foods contain hundreds of biologically active substances that work together to keep us healthy. Supplements may also be necessary, especially in the case of illness, but a healthy diet containing fruits and vegetables is critical. In addition, a vitamin obtained in pill form may not work the same in the human body, or it may not work at all, compared to the same vitamin found naturally in food.

## How Many Servings of Fruit and Vegetables Does a Person Need?

The American Heart Association and the American Cancer Society both recommend eating at least five servings of fruits and vegetables per day. When you consider that the average American only consumes three servings of fruits and vegetables a day (not counting potatoes, which are considered primarily a starch), five would be a good initial goal. Studies at Harvard University showed that each additional serving of fruits and vegetables reduced the risk of heart disease by 4 percent. The largest study to date, part of the Harvard-based Nurses' Health Study and Health Professionals' Follow-up Study, included over 110,000 people whose dietary and health habits were followed for 14 years. They found that people who consumed eight or more servings of fruits and vegetables per day were 30 percent less likely to have a heart attack or stroke than were those who consumed 1.5 servings of fruits and vegetables per day.

As a general rule, the more fruit and vegetables you eat the better. I recommend 7–12 servings each day. The Department of Health and Human Services (HHS) and the Department of Agriculture (USDA) recommend 9 servings of fruit and vegetables per day for men, and 7 for women. Before you get nervous about all these fruits and vegetables, let's make sure we're in agreement about servings.

## What Constitutes a "Serving?"

There are two simple ways to imagine the actual size of a "serving." Nutritionists describe a serving of a fruit or vegetable as being approximately the amount that can fit in the palm of your hand, or the amount found in a small glass of vegetable or fruit juice. Most Americans think of servings as being much larger than they are because of the way we use the word. It's easier than you think to get enough fruits and vegetables into your diet.

Before you begin to think that you might already be eating more servings than you thought because of the small size of a serving, remember that, despite what we consider the size of a serving, most Americans still consume only three servings per day of fruits and vegetables. If you are currently eating less than seven servings of fruits and vegetables per day, it's time to make some changes in your diet.

Let's consider what vitamins and minerals you need, especially if you have arthritis.

## Vitamin C—A Powerful Antioxidant

In the Framingham Osteoarthritis Cohort Study, which was part of the Framingham Heart Study that has yielded important information on the causes and prevention of heart disease, people who consumed a higher amount of vitamin C had a three-fold *lower* risk of cartilage loss and disease progression than people who took in less vitamin C.

A study in Britain involving more than 23,000 participants found that people who consumed less vitamin C had a higher risk of developing inflammatory polyarthritis, a form of rheumatoid arthritis that affects two or more joints. Reducing the risk of inflammatory polyarthritis may or may not correlate well with other types of arthritis, but the fact that vitamin C plays a positive role in protecting joints seems obvious.

Of note, a 2004 animal study showed that high levels of prolonged vitamin C intake actually *increase* the risk of arthritis progression in the knee. Human studies are needed to confirm or refute these results, but this does offer an argument to not exceed the recommended daily allowance (RDA), which is 90 mg for men and 75 mg for women. Because of this somewhat conflicting evidence, I do not recommend vitamin C supplementation for arthritis.

Eating fruits and vegetables that are loaded with vitamin C is an excellent approach to getting enough vitamin C and other important nutrients. Citrus fruits in general are excellent sources of vitamin C, including oranges (about 75 mg), guavas, grapefruit, pineapple, and kiwi fruit. Other good sources are broccoli, green peppers, tomatoes, sweet and white potatoes, watercress, and avocado.

## FAT-SOLUBLE AND WATER-SOLUBLE VITAMINS

Fat-soluble vitamins are absorbed in the small intestines. Once in the body, they are stored primarily in the liver and in fatty (adipose) tissues. The fat-soluble vitamins include A, D, E, and K. Extra care must be taken to not consume these vitamins in excess because they stay in the body longer and can more easily lead to toxicity. A well-balanced diet will not lead to toxicity, but vitamin supplementation might.

Water-soluble vitamins, including vitamins C and B, are excreted much more quickly than fat-soluble vitamins, and they need to be replaced more frequently.

# Vitamin E

Vitamin E is another powerful antioxidant. French scientists showed that 6 weeks of vitamin E supplementation in mice reduced the progression of bone and cartilage destruction, when compared with mice that were not given supplements.

## What Is an "International Unit"

An International Unit, or IU, is the amount of a certain substance that is required to produce a given effect. It is a way to standardize the amount of a given substance, such as a vitamin or mineral, without simply relying on weight.

German physicians showed that supplementation with 400 IU of vitamin E daily for 6 weeks reduced pain twice as much as a placebo. Another study found that 400 IU per day of vitamin E relieved arthritis pain symptoms more effectively than nonsteroidal anti-inflammatory drugs (NSAIDs), including aspirin, ibuprofen, and acetaminophen.

One part of the Framingham study showed that people who consumed 6–11 mg of vitamin E daily were significantly less likely to experience progression of arthritis of the knee than were people who consumed 2–5 mg. These dosages are much lower than usually given; vitamin E toxicity has been seen at doses of 3,000 IU per day for more than 7 weeks.

## A Note about Blood Thinners

The term "blood thinner" generally refers to drugs such as warfarin (Coumadin®), Plavix®, or aspirin, all of which have the property of reducing the clotting time of the blood and preventing the formation of blood clots. They are most commonly prescribed for people who have pre-existing cardiac conditions such as an arrhythmia or heart defect that increases your chances of developing such clots, which can lead to heart attacks, pulmonary embolisms, or strokes.

Some foods, including some of the supplements discussed in

this book, also act to reduce clotting time. If you are already taking a blood-thinning medication, this has the potential to cause problems.

If you are taking warfarin (Coumadin®), you already should be having a test regularly to make sure that the level of clotting is within the desired range. No foods or medications are specifically prohibited for people taking these medications. As has probably already been explained to you, the key is *consistency* in what foods you eat daily; the same applies to any changes in the vitamins or supplements that you take as part of an arthritis management program. A change in diet is compensated for by raising or lowering the dosage of the blood thinner. Therefore, if you change your intake of substances that have the potential to alter your clotting time, the dosage of blood thinner can be modified to reflect this.

---

A word of caution: If you are taking a blood thinner or other heart medications, you should take vitamin E only after discussing it with your doctor, because vitamin E acts as a blood thinner and can adversely affect the overall effects of your medications. In some studies, vitamin E adversely affected some patients with a history of heart problems, while others showed the reverse—that vitamin E actually has a protective effect on the heart.

The recommended daily allowance for vitamin E is 15–30 mg. I believe that people without a history of heart problems, and who are not taking a statin or blood-thinning medication, may consider taking 400 IU of vitamin E per day, with a recommendation from their doctor.

Foods that are rich in vitamin E include whole grains, spinach, broccoli, pumpkin, turnips, fish, poultry, lobster, and shrimp. As always, getting your vitamins from your diet is better than getting them from supplements.

## Vitamin A and Beta-Carotene

Vitamin A and beta-carotene are also important antioxidants that help prevent or counteract arthritis and inflammation. Beta-carotene is one of the *carotenoids*, antioxidant compounds that occur naturally in plants and give fruits and vegetables their color. People with low blood levels of beta-carotene have an increased risk of developing rheumatoid arthritis. This suggests that beta-carotene plays a role in maintaining joint health. The Framingham study showed that people who consumed more than 9,000 IU of beta-carotene daily had a reduced risk of arthritis development and progression, compared to those who consumed less than 5,000 IU.

Although most Americans consume less than 5,000 IU of beta-carotene daily, it is not hard to increase this to 9,000 IU by modifying your diet. For example, a single carrot has more than 20,000 IU. Other good sources of beta-carotene include pumpkin, broccoli, romaine lettuce, spinach, apricots, kale, collard greens, mangos, and papayas.

Beta-carotene supplements should be avoided, as they have been shown to be harmful for smokers, ex-smokers, and others. Large amounts, either in your diet or as supplements, can turn the soles of your feet or your palms orange. This discoloration is harmless, and will likely go away, but you should tell your doctor if this happens.

Vitamin A is important for healthy eyes, and a deficiency of vitamin A can lead to vision problems, but this important vitamin is also needed for skin, bone, and joint health. Too much vitamin A is dangerous. Symptoms may include skin problems, stomach problems, and/or weakness. Beta-carotene is a precursor of vitamin A, and if you consume foods rich in beta-carotene, you will have enough vitamin A in your diet.

## Vitamin D

Vitamin D is found primarily in foods to which vitamin D has been added ("fortified"). This vitamin is critical for bone health. Milk is usually fortified with vitamin D, but other dairy products such as cheese and ice cream generally are not. Calcium metabolism requires vitamin D, and it is also needed to maintain sufficient phosphorus levels in the blood. Other significant sources of dietary vitamin D include cod liver oil, tuna, salmon, fortified breakfast cereal, and eggs.

Vitamin D deficiency can result in rickets, a disease in which the bones become thin, brittle, and ultimately deformed. Rickets was much more common before fortifying milk with vitamin D began in the 1930s. Since then, rickets has been virtually eliminated. The other major source of vitamin D is the triggering of vitamin D synthesis in the skin by ultraviolet rays from the sun. Approximately 15 minutes of sun exposure daily will trigger a significant amount of vitamin D production. This moderate exposure will not cause damage from the sun. However, the skin becomes less and less effective at synthesizing vitamin D as we grow older, and many people are not exposed to sufficient sunlight during the winter months to produce a significant amount of vitamin D. I recommend 400 IU of vitamin D for everyone, increasing this to as much as 600 IU after the age of 70.

Participants in one study who had lower levels of vitamin D had up to a threefold increased risk of developing worsening arthritis of the knee, compared to those who consumed adequate amounts. Another study found that people with a lower intake of vitamin D had an increased risk of developing arthritis of the hip. Vitamin D is also critical in the prevention and treatment of osteoporosis. Toxicity is a concern and, if you take a supplement, don't take more than 1,000 IU per day.

Signs of toxicity may include constipation, stomach upset, backache, increased urination, increased blood pressure, cardiac arrhythmia, palpitations, and kidney stones. In children, appropriate dosages are lower, and even 400 IU per day may be toxic. It's a good idea to always speak with your doctor prior to starting any supplement program. If your doctor is not knowledgeable about supplements, consider seeing a nutritionist for assistance.

## BORON

Boron is a naturally occurring trace element found in soil, plants, and metal deposits. Trace elements are present in only very small amounts in the body. Despite their low concentrations, some organisms require trace elements to survive. In parts of the world where the soil and plants contain relatively small amounts of boron, arthritis is much more prevalent. Specifically, the incidence of arthritis is less than 10 percent in areas of the world where people consume 3–10 mg of boron per day.

In Israel, where dietary boron consumption is high thanks to an abundance of it in the soil, the incidence of arthritis is less than 1 percent. Boron intake is low in Jamaica and Mauritius, and arthritis rates there may be as high as 50–70 percent. Levels are also low in most of Australia. In contrast, Carnarvon in Western Australia has very high soil rates of boron, and the rate of arthritis is less than 1 percent. People come from as far as 1,000 miles away for months at a time to let "the climate" take away their arthritis symptoms, but it is probably the boron-rich food and water that have helped make Carnarvon the destination of choice for relieving arthritis symptoms.

Despite the apparent relationship between boron intake and arthritis, only one small controlled study has been published that firmly supports boron for managing arthritis symptoms. In 1990, twenty Australians with arthritis took either a placebo or 6 mg of boron per day for 8 weeks. Fifty percent of those who received boron reported an improvement in symptoms, as opposed to only

10 percent in those who received the placebo. As suggestive as this study was, the small sample size meant that it did not achieve "statistical significance," meaning that the researchers could not be sure their results were not due to chance. Unfortunately, definitive follow-up studies have not been reported, so we are left with this small, well-constructed experiment that yielded tantalizing but inconclusive data. However, it seems reasonable to include boron-rich foods in your diet. An additional advantage of adequate dietary boron consumption may be to help prevent calcium loss and bone demineralization.

Fruits, vegetables, and nuts are excellent sources of boron. Avocados are particularly rich in this element and contain approximately 2 mg per serving. Other excellent sources include almonds, dates, apples, green leafy vegetables, and raisins. A typical American diet provides between 1.5 and 3 mg of boron per day, but your daily dose of boron will increase effortlessly when you increase your daily consumption of fruits and vegetables.

Side effects from high dosages of boron (approximately 50 mg, which is difficult to achieve from diet alone) include nausea, vomiting, skin rashes, lethargy, and diarrhea. Concerns about the safety of boron, particularly when taken as a supplement, have been raised because in two small studies boron supplementation was found to increase the level of body estrogen, particularly in women already on estrogen-replacement therapy. Elevated estrogen levels increase the risk of breast and uterine cancer, and so there is a conceivable risk that boron supplementation may result in an increased risk of cancer. Other studies have shown that boron may increase testosterone levels, which is why boron is occasionally sold to bodybuilders as a way to help "pump up." One way or another, boron does seem to impact the body's hormonal balance. For these reasons, and because enough boron can be consumed from fruits and vegetables, I do not recommend taking boron supplements. Further research may change this view.

## Selenium

Selenium is another trace mineral that is important for overall good health. This powerful antioxidant helps the body recycle vitamin E, and it also helps other antioxidant enzymes to function properly and prevents cellular damage. Studies to date regarding selenium supplementation have been mixed, and no clinical human study definitively shows selenium supplements to be helpful for osteo-arthritis symptoms. For example, one study found that 200 mi-crograms of selenium per day taken for 3–6 months might reduce pain and joint inflammation in people with rheumatoid arthritis, while other studies have found no such link. Clearly, more studies are needed. However, because of its physiologic roles, it does seem reasonable to include foods containing selenium in your diet.

Good sources of selenium include salmon, tuna, shellfish, tur-key, whole wheat bread, and cottage cheese. Three ounces of tuna provide 95 percent of the daily recommended allowance of sele-nium. Brazil nuts have an unusually high amount—as much as 544 micrograms, or 780 percent of the recommended allowance. Eating them from time to time may be advisable, but I would not recommend eating them daily.

Symptoms of selenium toxicity can include nausea, vomiting, stomach pain, hair loss, garlic odor on the breath, and fatigue. The National Academy of Sciences recommends limiting your se-lenium intake to less than 400 micrograms per day for adults. I recommend eating 100–200 micrograms per day, as part of your diet, not as a supplement.

## Which Fruits and Vegetables Are Best?

Fruits and vegetables are loaded with antioxidants, which under-scores the importance of including them in your diet. But are all fruits and vegetables created equally? There are several ways to approach the issue of which fruits and vegetables are best. We have just reviewed some of the vitamins and minerals that are important to get from your diet, and which fruits and vegetables contain these nutrients. Another approach is to consider the merits of specific fruits and vegetables.

United States Department of Agriculture (USDA) researchers at Tufts University developed a laboratory test called the *Oxygen Radical Absorbance Capacity* (ORAC), to measure the antioxidant power in fruits, vegetables, and other foods. This test has become the "gold standard" for identifying which foods contain the most antioxidant power, meaning the food or nutrient that will remove the greatest number of harmful free radicals, thus protecting the body against free radical damage. However, there is one problem with this test. While some foods may have high amounts of anti-oxidants, not all of them are absorbed into the body. In technical terms, antioxidants may have different levels of *bioavailability* in our bodies. The ORAC test is therefore not perfect, because it does not tell us how much of the antioxidants we consume are actually available for use by the body.

The ORAC test has shown that blueberries have tremendous antioxidant power. One cup of wild, fresh blueberries has a Total Antioxidant Capacity (TAC) of 3,427, which is approximately ten times the USDA's recommendation.

Cultivated blueberries, cranberries, and blackberries are also high in antioxidants, followed closely by raspberries, strawberries, cherries, and grapes. The fruits that have the highest antioxidant levels are colored purple, blue, and red. Apples and orange-colored fruits such as navel oranges, peaches, and pineapples are also good sources of antioxidants.

When we use the word *antioxidants* in this context, we are talk-ing about the total antioxidant power in the *whole* food. This in-cludes vitamins A, C, E, the thousands of different flavonoids, and the many antioxidants that we have not yet identified but know

TABLE 7.1. *Foods and Their Antioxidant Levels*

| Food | Serving Size | Antioxidant Power (as measured by the ORAC test, TAC) |
| --- | --- | --- |
| Red beans | 1 cup | 27,454 |
| Wild blueberries | 1 cup | 13,427 |
| Cultivated blueberries | 1 cup | 9,019 |
| Cranberries | 1 cup | 8,983 |
| Artichoke hearts | 1 cup | 7,904 |
| Blackberries | 1 cup | 7,701 |
| Strawberries | 1 cup | 5,938 |
| Cherries | 1 cup | 4,873 |
| Red grapes | 1 cup | 2,016 |
| Green grapes | 1 cup | 1,789 |
| Red onion | 1 cup | 1834 |
| Orange | 1 fruit, 140g | 2,540 |
| Banana | 1 fruit, 118 g | 1,037 |
| Avocado | 1 fruit, 173 g | 3,344 |
| Granny apple | 1 fruit, 138 g | 5,381 |
| Broccoli, raw | 1 cup | 1,400 |
| Broccoli, cooked | 1 cup | 1,964 |

Table adapted from: http://www.vegparadise.com/news45.html

exist because of their ability to destroy free radicals. Dried and frozen fruits have much of the antioxidant power of fresh fruit, but you should avoid frozen fruit containing added sugar.

Vegetables also have antioxidant power, particularly artichoke hearts and leafy greens. Artichoke hearts are excellent, as is spinach, which appears to have an especially high bioavailability and may be one of the more powerful sources of antioxidants. Other vegetables containing a large amount of antioxidants include Brussels sprouts, kale, asparagus, onions, red cabbage, broccoli, and eggplant. Beans, red beans in particular, are also excellent sources of antioxidants. In fact, there are twice as many antioxidants in a cup of small red beans as there are in a cup of wild blueberries.

Fruits and vegetables are also excellent sources of fiber. Most of us do not eat enough fiber. Eating more fiber will reduce your risk of constipation, help cleanse toxins from your colon, reduce potential discomfort, and help your body absorb the important nutrients you are consuming.

## Preparing Fruit and Vegetables

Raw foods retain all of their antioxidant power, but not everyone enjoys raw fruits and vegetables. Thus, it is important to know what happens to the antioxidants in fruits and vegetables when they are steamed, broiled, fried, boiled, and grilled. For example, raw asparagus has 25 percent more antioxidant power than steamed asparagus.

How should fruits and vegetables be prepared so that they retain the most antioxidant power possible, taste great, and are safe to eat?

First, always wash your hands before handling fruits and vegetables; also wash the surface of the fruit or vegetable. As a general rule, antioxidants are lost when the food is exposed to heated water for prolonged periods of time. Steaming is the best cooking method for vegetables because it minimizes the loss of nutrients. Conversely, steaming sometimes *increases* the antioxidant power of a food. For example, steamed red cabbage has more than twice the amount of antioxidant power of raw red cabbage. Although steaming is usually the best cooking option, remember that boiled vegetables are better than no vegetables.

Another way to minimize potential antioxidant loss during cooking is to cut the food into large rather than small pieces. This minimizes the surface area of the food that is exposed to the cooking process, and may save more antioxidants.

## TIPS FOR INCREASING FRUIT AND VEGETABLE INTAKE:

- Eat a new fruit or vegetable every day.

- Always have a bowl of fruit or vegetables in the refrigerator for snacks. It's easy to eat a small bowl of chopped broccoli or plum tomatoes while working, before dinner, or even while watching television.

- Some people eat only fruit in the morning, which seems to stop their craving for coffee and sweets. Check with your doctor first, but for many people this is a good alternative.

- Eat vegetable soup.

- Challenge yourself to see how many different colored fruits and vegetables you can eat in a day.

- A juicer is a good way to get a few extra servings of fruit and vegetables. Try making a smoothie with low-fat ice cream.

- Bring a zip-locked bag of vegetables with you to work and snack on them during the day.

Science is not ready to state definitively which individual fruits and vegetables are better than others. Therefore, eating a healthy mix is probably the best way to ensure that you get all of the antioxidants, vitamins, minerals, and other nutrients that your body requires for optimal health. This is also your best chance of reducing inflammation and relieving your arthritis symptoms.

# 8

# Eat More Cold-Water Fish

IN THE 1950s and 1960s, thanks in large part to the Framingham Heart Study, medical researchers began to understand that increased fat consumption is associated with a higher risk of heart disease. Researchers were surprised, however, when they found in the early 1970s that some groups of people had a low incidence of heart disease despite having a diet based primarily on fat. For example, the natives of western Greenland had a very low incidence of heart disease. Danes living in the same area had significantly higher rates of cardiovascular disease than the native Greenlanders. The major difference between the two groups was their diets. The Danes maintained a typical European diet, which was rich in saturated fat and cholesterol from meat and dairy products, while the natives obtained their fats from fish, whales, walrus, and seals, which are rich in omega-3 fatty acids. These same findings were seen in the Nunavik Inuit of Quebec, whose fish-based diet was associated with a 50 percent lower mortality rate, compared to their neighbors.

## WHAT ARE OMEGA-3 FATTY ACIDS?

Long-chain fatty acids are a major component of the walls of the cells of the body. It is important that these walls be pliable, because hard, rigid walls make for unhealthy cells. The more flexible the cell wall, the more able it is for the cell to communicate with other cells, and for it to allow important proteins and nutrients to pass through its membranous surface. There are different kinds of fatty acids, but the two main types that are discussed here are omega-3 and omega-6. The difference between them on a molecular level is simply the placement of a single carbon bond. However, this small difference results in omega-3 fatty acids being *hydrophilic*, meaning that they accept water into their structure more readily than omega-6 fatty acids. This makes them more flexible and pliable. The ratio between these two types of fatty acids in the foods we eat has a profound impact on how our cells function, and subsequently on how healthy we are.

Two specific fatty acids are considered essential, because our bodies don't manufacture them and they must be obtained from food. *Linoleic acid* is an omega-6 fatty acid that we get ample amounts of in our diet. In fact, while we need to eat some linoleic acid, most of us consume far too much of it. The other essential fatty acid is *alpha-linolenic acid*, one of three omega-3 fatty acids. Alpha-linolenic acid is converted by the body into the two other omega-3 fatty acids: eicosapentaenoic acid (EPA) and docosahexaenoic acid (DHA). Raw nuts, seeds, and legumes, and unsaturated vegetable oils such as borage, grape seed, primrose, sesame, and soybean are healthful sources of omega-6 fatty acids.

## The Effects of Fatty Acids in the Body

Too much omega-6 and not enough omega-3 fatty acids in the cells of the heart make the tissue less pliable, and therefore the heart is less efficient at pumping. In addition, they are believed to contribute to arteriosclerosis, so that the heart has to pump harder to move the blood through the arteries and to the organs. This extra effort causes blood pressure to rise. Reversing this process is believed to be one of the ways in which a diet rich in omega-3 fatty acids and low in omega-6 fatty acids may lower blood pressure.

Platelets, the cells in your blood vessels that are responsible for clotting, are one of the primary culprits in the development of cholesterol plaques in the arteries, which leads to coronary artery disease, heart disease, and heart attacks. Omega-3 fatty acids in the membrane also help platelets move through the arteries without sticking together. By allowing them to slip and slide past each other—thanks to the malleable cell membranes—a diet rich in omega-3 fatty acids is believed to lower the risk of heart disease.

Omega-6 fatty acids are also *proinflammatory*, because they are broken down by the body and converted into prostaglandins and other inflammatory proteins. These proteins cause inflammation. In fact, steroids and nonsteroidal anti-inflammatory drugs (NSAIDs), such as ibuprofen and naproxen, work by blocking the formation of these same inflammatory proteins.

Omega-3 fatty acids are also converted into inflammatory proteins, but this conversion takes place much more slowly, so that the body's natural mechanisms of breaking down inflammatory mediators occur before inflammation has a chance to take place. When you consume omega-6 fatty acids, inflammatory proteins are built so quickly that the body's natural process of metabolizing them is overwhelmed, and inflammation and its symptoms are much more likely to occur. Unchecked inflammation may be a factor in the development of a number of diseases, including heart disease. Obviously, ingesting substances that create more inflammatory proteins in the body is not good for people struggling with arthritis.

## Balancing Fatty Acids

How much of your diet should come from omega-3, and how much from omega-6 fatty acids? The rate of converting the consumed fatty acids into the membranes of the cells of the body, and the rate of metabolizing the fatty acids and building them into inflammatory mediators, is averaged out over the different kinds of fatty acids you eat. The problem is not whether or not you consume too much omega-6 fatty acids, but rather the *ratio* of omega-6 to omega-3 fatty acids in your diet.

From an evolutionary standpoint, humans historically sustained themselves on diets rich in seafood, nuts, vegetables, and grass-fed game, all of which are rich in omega-3 fatty acids. Scientists generally believe that humans are designed to function optimally when the food they consume has a ratio of omega-6 to omega-3 fatty acids of 1:1 or 2:1, but no higher than 4:1. The average American diet has a ratio of 10-30:1, or even higher, which is not healthy. This situation probably developed as the result of our increasing consumption of processed food, which contains a high amount of hydrogenated oil. This wildly skewed ratio has been blamed for contributing to and perhaps being the cause of heart disease, a leading cause of death in the United States.

## HYDROGENATED AND NON-HYDROGENATED OILS

When oils are hydrogenated—a process that makes the oil more solid, as is commonly done in the production of margarine—the linoleic acid is converted into trans-fatty acids, which are harmful to the body. Highly processed foods, such as potato chips, cookies, some ice cream, fast food, and packaged and canned foods, contain large amounts of hydrogenated oils in order to extend shelf life. These foods should be eaten sparingly or eliminated entirely from your diet.

It is extremely important that you change your eating habits to have a more balanced ratio of omega-6 to omega-3 fatty acids. The ratio should be 4:1 or less, but I recommend a ratio of no more than 2:1 for most people, in order to reduce the risk of heart disease, cancer, diabetes, depression, and arthritis. Exceptions to this include people with bleeding disorders and/or a history of bleeding, and people who are taking blood thinners. Always discuss the options with your physician before changing your diet. A consultation with a nutritionist in conjunction with your physician would also be very helpful.

## WHICH FOODS CONTAIN OMEGA-3 FATTY ACIDS?

Fish are the best single source of omega-3 fatty acids. If you're not allergic to fish, and are neither a vegetarian nor a vegan, you need to consider the important, life-saving qualities of fish. It is high in protein, low in overall fat, high in omega-3 fatty acids, and high in B-vitamins, minerals, and even calcium.

There are other ways to get enough omega-3 fatty acids if you are a vegetarian or simply don't like fish. Vegetable oils are rich in omega-3 fatty acids, including primrose, canola, linseed, walnut, ground or milled flaxseed, and wheat germ oils. Other foods rich in omega-3 fatty acids include walnuts, pumpkin seeds, hemp seeds, tofu, green leafy vegetables, soybeans, certain margarines, grass-fed game, and chickens that are fed omega-3 fatty acids and the yolks of their eggs. However, there is some evidence that the alpha-linolenic acid consumed in green leafy vegetables and sources other than fish are not metabolized into EPA and DHA omega-3 fatty acids as readily as when alpha-linolenic acid is consumed in fish.

Another way to make sure you have enough "good" fatty acids in your diet is with olive oil, which contains large amounts of an omega-9 fatty acid called *oleic acid*. Omega-9 fatty acids are less well studied than omega-3 fatty acids, but they are metabolized into icosatrienoic acid (ETA), which competes with omega-6 fatty acids in the same way that omega-3 fatty acids compete with them for metabolism, incorporation into the cell membranes, and the formation of painful and dangerous inflammatory proteins.

Mediterranean populations consume large amounts of olive oil, and the "Mediterranean diet" has been gaining popularity in America. Some scientists have suggested that the lower incidence of arthritis in Mediterranean populations may be a result of the amount of omega-9 fatty acid they consume via olive oil.

One study of rheumatoid arthritis patients showed that people who consumed 6 g/day of olive oil in capsule form experienced a significant improvement in their arthritis symptoms after 6 months. Many of the participants who consumed olive oil were able to reduce their NSAID use. Other studies have also found a correlation between increased olive oil consumption and reduced risk of developing rheumatoid arthritis.

Because of the inflammatory component that we now know exists in osteoarthritis, it is reasonable and perhaps likely that an anti-inflammatory diet including olive oil could decrease the severity of arthritis symptoms and disease progression.

## Fish and Mercury

As you have probably read in news reports, the mercury present in some fish can affect the human brain, spinal cord, liver, and kidneys. Mercury is naturally present in the environment in low levels, but industrial pollution has resulted in large amounts ending up in our lakes, rivers, and oceans. Microorganisms in the water convert the mercury into highly toxic methyl mercury, which is then eaten by small fish. Because larger fish eat the smaller ones, methyl mercury levels are highest in larger, predatory fish.

The Food and Drug Administration (FDA) limits the amount of mercury allowed in fish sold for human consumption to 1 part per million (ppm) of mercury. According to the FDA surveys of 1990-2003, shark has 0.99 ppm mercury, swordfish 0.97 ppm, orange roughy 0.54 ppm, canned albacore tuna 0.35 ppm, canned light tuna 0.12 ppm, and trout and salmon each have less than 0.1 ppm.

Because fetuses and young children are particularly vulnerable to the effects of mercury, it is particularly important that children younger than five, pregnant women, women who may become pregnant, and nursing mothers closely monitor and limit their potential mercury consumption. People in these groups should limit their weekly fish and shellfish consumption to 12 ounces or less of canned light tuna, shrimp, and salmon.

The FDA recommends that people who are not in these groups limit their consumption of large predatory fish to one serving per week. Fish with levels of about 0.5 ppm (such as orange roughy) should be limited to two servings per week. The FDA does not believe it is necessary to limit weekly consumption of the top ten seafood species currently on the market: canned tuna, shrimp, salmon, clams, cod, pollock, flatfish, crabs, and scallops, because their mercury is less than 0.2 ppm.

Farm-raised fish are generally less expensive than wild fish, but they tend to have more calories and fat, and less protein. They also tend to contain a higher level of toxins because of the food they are usually fed. You should therefore eat wild fish whenever possible.

## Putting It All Together

- ▶ Eat small, cold-water fish, such as wild salmon and light canned tuna, 2–4 times per week.
- ▶ Use oils rich in omega-3 fatty acids, such as flaxseed, canola, olive, and primrose seed.

▶ Cut down on processed foods and animal fat that contain proinflammatory omega-6 fatty acids.

▶ Aim for a ratio of omega-6 to omega-3 fatty acids consumption of 2:1, and be sure that it does not exceed 4:1.

▶ Eat green leafy vegetables and tofu to supplement your omega-3 fatty acid consumption.

▶ If you have no contraindications, and after a discussion with your physician, take fish oil, evening primrose seed oil, flax-seed oil, or borage seed oil supplements.

# 9

# Eat Red Meat Sparingly

WHEN I was selected as a finalist for a research award at a national conference in 2005, I called my wife, who immediately said, "Let's celebrate! Where do you want to go?"

I knew the answer to her question right away, and so did she: a local restaurant that had terrific, mouth-watering, juicy, makes you feel like you were in Omaha and had just come in from a cattle drive, prime rib.

If you don't care for red meat, or you are a vegetarian or a vegan, this chapter is not for you. If anything, read it and be thankful that you are already one step closer to a healthy diet without having to work at it. For all my fellow meat-lovers, it is with great empathy that I inform you that the amount of meat in your future will be less—or at least it should be.

## WHY SHOULD I EAT LESS RED MEAT?

A maximum of two servings a week of red meat is recommended, and they should be limited to 3 ounces a serving, roughly the size of a deck of cards. Red meat and processed meats have been linked to a variety of cancers. The strongest link appears to be with colorectal cancer. People who eat substantial amounts of red meat have twice the risk of suffering from colorectal cancer than those who eat less. Other types of cancer associated with eating meat include renal, breast, pancreatic, and prostate cancer. Undoubtedly, eating larger amounts puts you at significantly greater risk for suffering from heart disease. One study found that men who ate beef four or more times per week were twice as likely to die from heart disease as men who did not eat beef.

One of the biggest myths in this country is that women don't get heart disease. Heart disease is a major killer of men and women, but women are more likely to die from a heart attack than men. This is due to a multitude of factors, including a variety of less predictable initial symptoms in women. Men and women need to be equally concerned with their diets for a variety of reasons.

Eating more red meat also increases proinflammatory proteins. Red meat is rich in omega-6 fatty acids, which, as we noted in the last chapter, are broken down into the proinflammatory proteins that people with arthritis need to avoid. When you have arthritis and eat red meat, you increase the possibility of inflammation and make it more likely that you will need medications.

One research study in Britain found that increased red meat consumption was associated with as much as a two-fold increased risk of developing rheumatoid arthritis. This study did not provide a direct relationship between red meat and osteoarthritis, and other factors such as general protein consumption, may have been involved. If there is a causal relationship between red meat and rheumatoid arthritis, it is probably associated with the collagen in red meat, or perhaps some other substance that triggers an immune response.

In conclusion, there is the potential for red meat to produce and exacerbate the symptoms associated with any type of arthritis, including rheumatoid arthritis and osteoarthritis, as well as related problems such as gout. In addition to its other medical benefits, reducing your red meat consumption will also reduce the inflammatory proteins circulating in your body and help alleviate your arthritis-related pain and inflammation.

# 10.

## Processed Foods

PROCESSING TECHNOLOGY can rid food of dangerous, even deadly bacteria such as certain virulent strains of *E. coli* and *Salmonella* and, in some cases, processing foods may make them more nutritious. Lycopene, for example, is a powerful antioxidant found in tomatoes. Converting tomatoes to tomato paste may actually increase the amount of lycopene available to the body. Processed cereals, breads, and other foods usually contain added vitamins and minerals. We can add vitamins to all of our breakfast, lunch, and dinner foods. We can add fiber to fat-filled spreads to limit cholesterol. These are all positive developments.

However, taken to the extreme, they can also send a dangerous signal.

A problem arises when we begin to think that we can manipulate food to the point of no longer relying on natural foods. A cereal bar packed with vitamins and minerals and eaten as a "meal replacement" is not inherently a bad thing. It's certainly convenient and may help some people improve their nutrition and lose extra weight. However, no cereal bar can replace the nutrients found in a healthy salad made with fruits or vegetables. Food processing is best when it seeks to *enhance* Nature's foods, rather than try to replace them.

The processed foods that are best avoided are the sugary kind.

Candies, chocolates, ice cream, and all the rest of the junk food that we eat too much of are full of sugar and saturated fats, and they greatly contribute to the obesity epidemic in America. Reducing, moderating, and ultimately even eliminating your intake of sweets will help you to lose weight and maintain a healthy weight, while reducing fat and increasing lean muscle. In the end, you will feel better both psychologically and physically.

Cutting down on processed foods in favor of eating more fruits and vegetables will also help give you the anti-inflammatory edge you need to break the cycle of pain and inflammation in your joints.

# 11

# Changing Your Diet: Turning Words into Action

How do you go from eating two slices of pizza and a bowl of ice cream to eating a bowl of fruit salad, a side dish of vegetables, tuna, and a glass of low-fat milk? If you want to be successful in the long run, the answer is *slowly*. Prepare yourself to take the steps necessary to change your diet, so you can stay with the changes you make.

Knowledge is the first step. Having read the preceding chapters, you now understand which foods are good for you and which ones are not. With this knowledge comes the responsibility to make informed decisions about the food you eat. The amazing thing about changing any lifestyle habit is that it can be profoundly difficult or amazingly easy—it all depends on your frame of mind. The good thing is that your frame of mind is completely up to you. Just because you had a negative attitude toward making healthy lifestyle choices in the past doesn't mean you must have the same negative attitudes in the present. *You* are in control.

Here's how to get started:

Remember that your ultimate goal is to eat a healthy diet. This doesn't mean it has to be completely healthy tomorrow or the next day, or even the day after. The more gradually you change your diet, the more likely you are to stick with the changes. If you had pizza every night for dinner until today, try eating a fruit salad before having pizza tomorrow, not necessarily instead of pizza. Instead of two slices, have one slice. The next night, have a vegetable platter and a bowl of tuna salad. If you're still hungry, have part of a slice of pizza, and so forth. By incorporating small changes into your diet over a few weeks, you will soon find that you are making big changes and enjoying them. The best anecdote I can give is a personal one:

I used to love eating sweets, chips, ice cream, and pizza. Clearly, I had to make some changes. The first one I made was to start drinking more water and all-natural, 100 percent juice. I soon realized that I wasn't as hungry, and I had more energy. Next, I started keeping fruit and vegetable snacks close by. I began to snack on plum tomatoes instead of potato chips while writing at the computer. I ate veggies instead of sugary snacks at lunch. I soon started to crave a bowl of carrots as much as I had once craved a package of M&Ms™. I wasn't having the highs and lows that resulted from my blood sugar levels rising and falling. I also began to appreciate that often I ate a snack not because I was hungry, but because the physical act of sitting and munching on something gave me a mental break from what I was doing. For example, while writing, I used to get up and go to the kitchen and pull out a bag of chips. I would sit at the kitchen table or pace around the room and munch. The break allowed my mind to relax and wander, almost like a form of meditation.

An important step for me was freeing myself from associating taking a break with eating. I began to take breaks without the pretense of hunger. Sometimes I would drink a glass of water or juice, and eat a few plum tomatoes. Other times I would go for a brisk walk. Sometimes I would simply sit in a comfortable chair by a window and watch the birds in the trees for a few minutes. Without the chips and all of the accompanying saturated fats flowing through my blood, I returned to my writing feeling more refreshed.

As I learned to significantly cut down on sweets and ice cream, my final hurdle was red meat and pizza. To my delight and surprise, I found them relatively easy to give up. In the first place, as I ate more fruits and vegetables, and kept better hydrated, my body began to detoxify. When I occasionally ate a bag of chips or a bowl of ice cream, I felt physically bad—not guilty. Eating chips and sweets made me feel sluggish, and I no longer craved them. Likewise, a heavy meal of steak or fried food was no longer quite so satisfying. As I began to substitute more small cold-water fish for steaks and hamburgers, I found myself wanting more fish and less red meat. Pizza, too, seemed heavy and not as appetizing.

As I ate healthier food and stayed better hydrated, I felt better, had more energy, and wanted to continue to keep the natural high that these habits produced. I was also exercising more, and this, too, made me feel better and have more energy. I reconnected with my core value of staying healthy. As we will discuss later, once we identify our core values, it is easier to act in accordance with them. By identifying *staying healthy* as a core value, it was easier for me to make healthier choices. When confronted with a slice of pizza or a hamburger, the choice I had to make wasn't, "How hungry am I?" or "Do I deserve this special food?" Instead, the choice was simply, "Is eating this food consistent with my core value of staying healthy?" Since I knew that eating healthy was integral to staying healthy, I chose not to have the fatty food.

Of course, I allowed myself indulgences, particularly in the beginning. Once in a while I decided that I really wanted that pizza, candy, or ice cream, but I would have less than usual, and I would remind myself it was a treat. While breaking my new diet, I concentrated not on how good the pizza tasted, but rather on how it really wasn't as satisfying as I had once thought. It tasted good, but not *that* good. And, certainly, hamburger tasted no better than my baked tilapia with a side of steamed spinach and fresh tomatoes.

Slowly, I began to realize I no longer wanted to eat junk food.

That's when I realized I wasn't dieting anymore. I had simply adopted a healthier diet that I preferred because of the way it made me feel. I had learned to enjoy the new and wonderful tastes I was experiencing.

How do you change your frame of mind and decide it's time to take better care of yourself?

Before making a change, you have to know what's important to you. You need to know your inner-self—what drives you and what your core values are.

No one can identify your core values for you; only you can do this. They might include being good to your family, working hard, or spending time with your children and grandchildren. They might be about being trustworthy, striving for excellence, or being dependable. Hopefully, one of your core values will be staying healthy.

When you are faced with a decision about what to eat, consider whether or not eating that particular food is consistent with your core values. Is eating a bag of salty potato chips consistent with staying healthy? Once you've identified your core values and have committed to them, making the right choices will become much easier, and eventually the right choices will become automatic.

You can't completely change your diet overnight, and making slower changes will provide more lasting results. If you are truly committed, there is no rush, because your goal is a lifelong change in eating habits. It's also okay to have occasional setbacks. In fact, I would encourage you to listen to your cravings. If they become overwhelming, consider eating a small amount of the food you crave.

As your eating pattern improves and you start to exercise, when you do give in to your cravings, you will find that you relish the abandoned food more from an emotional and nostalgic association than because of its taste. Think about whether it's really as good as you remember; chances are that it won't be. Gradually leave the fatty, salty, sugary foods behind in favor of a healthier diet. You will feel better, and you will be acting in keeping with your core value of staying healthy.

If you want to make healthy changes in your eating behavior, but are having difficulty, the strategies provided in *Living Smart: Five Essential Skills to Change Your Health Habits Forever* (DiaMedica, 2008) will help you develop the habits your need to make your diet a success.

# PART III:

## Exercise

EXERCISE IS an important part of arthritis treatment and prevention. This section discusses the principles of exercising, which exercises are right for each individual, and how to do them. Exercise is closely related to the third rule of arthritis management:

**Rule #3:** Joints require movement to restore function and maintain optimal health.

Joints degenerate if you don't exercise them. As discussed in earlier chapters, without movement, your joints will not receive sufficient nourishment because they do not have a direct blood supply. The cartilage will begin to erode, the shock-absorbing capacity of the joints will diminish, and the supporting ligaments and muscles will weaken. Your joints will feel stiff and hurt when you need them to support you. What's the good news? By exercising, you can nourish and strengthen your joints, and reduce your pain and stiffness. It's never too late to start exercising.

Until the last 20–30 years, the prevailing thought was that the best treatment for arthritis was rest. This seemed reasonable, but we now know it was wrong. Research has unequivocally demonstrated that exercise, when done correctly, actually reduces the pain and stiffness associated with arthritis. For example, a Tufts University study showed that 43 percent of older men and women with moderate-to-severe arthritis of the knee were able to increase muscle strength and decrease pain and disability after completing a strength training program. Other studies have also shown decreased pain, stiffness, and disability using a variety of exercise regimens.

Exercise can help prevent arthritis by stretching and strengthening the structures surrounding the joints, as well as helping to keep the joints well nourished. In addition, exercise helps you lose weight, which is another way to reduce your risk for developing arthritis. Obesity also increases the pain and disability associated with arthritis, and the combination of obesity and arthritis are ingredients for a potentially devastating cycle.

Understanding why you need to exercise is a good place to start. In the next chapter, we'll talk about the principles of exercise.

## THE MANY BENEFITS OF EXERCISE

In addition to alleviating the symptoms of arthritis, exercise has been shown to:

- Increase life span
- Decrease heart disease
- Decrease the incidence of diabetes
- Decrease depression and anxiety
- Decrease body fat
- Lower blood pressure
- Decrease the risk of developing certain types of cancers
- Decrease the risk of osteoporosis and slow its progression
- Potentially decrease the risk of developing certain gastrointestinal problems such as ulcers, indigestion, constipation, and diverticulosis
- Increase self-esteem and self-confidence

# 12

# General Exercise Principles: Getting Started

THE THREE basic components of exercise are aerobic conditioning, strength training, and flexibility. Any exercise program that does not incorporate all three is incomplete. However,
no single exercise prescription will fit everyone. Furthermore, any
good exercise program should change and evolve over time to fit
your changing needs. Your physician can perform a general exam
to make sure it is safe for you to exercise and tell you how strenu-
ously you can safely exercise. A physical medicine and rehabilitation doctor, also called a *physiatrist*, often works closely with physical therapists to design specific exercise prescriptions to meet the
needs of individuals, so they can be sure to get the most out of their
exercise routine.

## GET A MEDICAL CHECK-UP FIRST

Always check with your doctor before beginning any new exercise
regimen to make sure you are medically able to participate. Only
your doctor can determine how much exercise is safe for you.
Starting an exercise program that is more strenuous than you are
ready for can result in injury and serious medical problems.

## FLEXIBILITY

Having stressed the importance of medical supervision, let's discuss some of the basic principles of any exercise program. The first is *flexibility*, which is determined by the range of motion you have in any given joint. Maintaining good flexibility is essential, particularly if you have arthritis. Some Eastern cultures understand how important this is, and measure a person's age not in years but in lost flexibility.

Flexibility exercises should be performed before and after strength training exercises. If they are done before strength training, they should follow a 5–10 minute warm-up period, which increases blood flow to your muscles so you can get a good stretch. Without the warm-up, your stretching may result in injury when you try to stretch tight muscles. Your warm-up can be a brisk walk or other brief aerobic exercise, or a combination of light aerobic exercise and light weight training such as lifting a 5-pound dumbbell. The important part of any warm-up is to get your heart pumping a little faster than baseline and your blood flowing.

To increase your strength, you need to push your muscles to work past their comfort zone. Generally speaking, the harder you push your muscles, the stronger they will become. Similarly, you must overstretch to a certain extent to increase your flexibility. This is one of the reasons warming up is so important. However, stretching should never be painful—a painful stretch means that you have gone too far. Strength training can cause some pain in the muscles, but it should never be painful in the joints. If a joint hurts while strength training, back off until it stops hurting. If you are unsure if it is the joint or the muscle that is hurting, stop what you are doing and ask your doctor.

## Aerobic Conditioning

Aerobic conditioning is vital to any comprehensive training program. There are many good ways to get a good aerobic workout. Weight-bearing exercises that do not put increased stress across your joints are the best. Running is one example of a weight-bearing exercise, but it puts a lot of stress on the joints. Using an elliptical machine at the gym is a good compromise because it is weight-bearing but easier on the joints. In the end, the aerobic training program that is right for you will be one that you enjoy and do consistently.

## Join the Gym

Consider joining a gym or health club. There is no absolute right or wrong when it comes to whether or not you should belong to a gym. Every individual is different. However, you should at least consider it. Some potential advantages of joining a gym include:

- ▶ It gets you out of the house and can be a positive social experience.
- ▶ Gyms and health clubs usually have better equipment and more workout space than you have at home.
- ▶ It is easier to find a trainer at most gyms.
- ▶ Many people find that the commitment to go to the gym each day makes it easier for them to actually work out on a daily basis. By contrast, a commitment to working out at home can be put off indefinitely with excuses ranging from "I'll go downstairs and work out right after this television show" to "I'll do it after dinner." Once you're home and surrounded by your loved ones and a million distractions, it may be harder to push yourself to work out. If you have a treadmill, ski-track,

exercise bike, or other piece of exercise equipment gathering dust in a corner or closet, you know what I'm talking about.

► Your health club might have classes that you enjoy.

► The gym might have a heated pool. Many people with arthritis find that aquatic exercises are helpful. They are easier on the joints because the water buoys the body. Plus, it feels good.

There are also potential negatives to joining a gym, including:

► You may not live close to a good facility.

► A gym membership can be expensive, though there are reasonably priced gyms in most areas.

► Some people are embarrassed about their bodies, or about not being able to keep up with other people in their exercise classes.

## SELF-IMAGE AT THE GYM

Gyms can be intimidating places for many people. Advertisements on television classically show superbly toned models performing exercises with professional athleticism. When you look in the mirror, you may think to yourself, "I don't fit in there," but remember, you are exercising for *you* and not for the other people in the gym. Be proud of yourself and your commitment to improving your health. Consider, too, that your fear may melt away when you actually go to the gym and realize that most of the people there don't look like the people in the commercials either. Sometimes, once you immerse yourself in any challenge, including exercising, fear and insecurity will no longer be an issue. However, if your feelings keep you from going or cause you serious distress, you should consider other alternatives.

A gentle course of yoga or tai chi that focuses on excellent form and is practiced on a regular basis can be immensely helpful. As always, get clearance from your doctor first, and make sure you practice the movements under the guidance of an experienced professional. Yoga, in particular, can be dangerous if you push too far too fast.

Ideally, after you get medical clearance to participate in a given exercise program, your physician will write a detailed physical therapy program for you to participate in. In this case, you will meet with a physical therapist 2–3 times a week until you feel comfortable doing the exercises on your own. As an alternative, find a personal trainer to show you how to perform the exercises that are right for you. Once you are comfortable with your exercise routine, check periodically with your therapist or trainer to make sure you are doing the exercises correctly. Also explore new exercises to keep your routine fresh and engaging.

# 13

# Stretching

EVERYONE CAN and should stretch, although many people are initially reluctant to begin a stretching regimen. They say things like: "Oh, I've always been tight. I don't need to stretch. It's just how I'm built. I'm not flexible."

In fact, nothing could be further from the truth, although everyone has limitations. A 60-year-old man, who has never stretched before and can barely bend over and touch his knees, let alone his toes, is unlikely to ever become a competitive gymnast or yoga master. However, he can and should improve his flexibility. Even a modest improvement in flexibility can have a profound impact on joint problems.

If you have never stretched before, I encourage you to make a commitment to it. Start slowly, under the direction of an experienced physician, physical therapist, or trainer. After a few weeks, you will become more flexible, which should help you control and alleviate your arthritis symptoms.

Stretching all of your muscles will treat any pain you already have, and it will help ensure that you don't develop pain somewhere else, so do as much of a whole-body workout as you can. Emphasizing certain stretching exercises based on your specific needs is good common sense. For example, if you have tight hamstrings, but very flexible hip flexors and quadriceps, stretch your hip flexors and quadriceps less and your hamstrings more.

Problems can arise if you don't pay attention to the *kinetic chain* that connects all the parts of your body. For example, a force that acts on your feet will be felt in your knees, hips, lower back, and upper back. If your knee hurts, and you only stretch and strengthen the muscles around it, you may improve slightly, but you will not get the same effect as you would if you addressed your entire body. Consider the following scenario. Jim has left knee pain. His doctor does some tests and tells him it's okay to exercise. The doctor gives Jim exercises to stretch and strengthen his quadriceps and hamstrings. These are the primary muscles that work directly on the knee; the quadriceps extends the knee and the hamstrings flex it. However, what if Jim's hip flexors are tight?

When one component of your biomechanics is altered, the rest will follow. For example, if Jim is an average middle-aged man, his hip flexors are probably tight and pull his upper pelvis forward, which alters his center of gravity and movement. To compensate, his lower back has to overextend backward—this is one of the reasons that tight hip flexors so often contribute to lower back pain. Increased pressure is placed on parts of the knee that are not designed to cushion the increased loads. The end result is that, despite stretching the immediate muscles around the knee, increased stress will continue to be placed on the knee simply because the hip flexors were not stretched.

To a lesser extent, tight shoulders place stress on the upper back, which is transmitted to the lower back and, in turn, to the hips, knees, and ankles. The further a joint is from the affected joint, the less the probable impact, but there will still be some. If you have a painful lower extremity joint, such as the hip, knee, or ankle, you need to stretch the entire lower extremity on both sides of your body as well as your lower back. To a lesser extent, it's important to stretch your upper back and arms.

Finally, if you only stretch your right side because that's the side that is painful, your left side will become tighter. This asymmetry will create tension on your spine, muscles, and other joints, ultimately leading to worsening biomechanics, chronic stress, and pain. Therefore, it is important to stretch and strengthen both sides of your body as evenly and symmetrically as possible.

## Hold That Stretch

Hold each of the following stretch positions for at least 20 full seconds and then return slowly to the starting position. Repeat this 3 times per stretching exercise for each side of the body. Remember to continue breathing in a smooth, controlled manner throughout the stretch. Don't hold your breath. If you are new to stretching, it is also advisable to do these stretches in front of a mirror. Once you have internalized the correct body placement for each of the stretches, you will be able to do them comfortably.

These stretches were selected after reviewing hundreds of different exercises. Always discuss which exercises may be best for you with a qualified professional. If you are unsure about how to do any of the exercises, don't do them. If you feel pain, stop and discuss your options with your physician, physical therapist, or trainer.

## The Stretches

▸ **Neck:**

Place your right hand over your head so that it rests on your left ear (Figure 13.1A). Gently and slowly, pull your head so that your right ear comes to rest on your right shoulder (Figure 13.1B). Hold the pose for 20 seconds. Return to the starting position and repeat the stretch, this time pulling your left ear to your left shoulder. Hold for 20 seconds. Return to starting position. Repeat this 3 times.

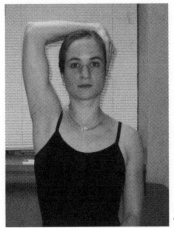

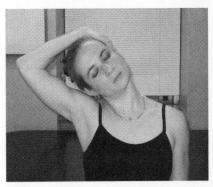

13.1B

13.1A

Turn your head so that you are looking over your left shoulder. You may use your left hand to help gently push your chin in the direction of your left shoulder (Figure 13.2). Feel a gentle stretch. Hold the pose for 20 seconds. Return slowly to the starting position and repeat to the right side. Hold for 20 seconds. Repeat this 3 times.

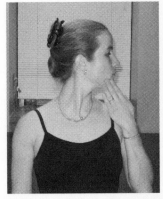

13.2

▶ **Shoulders:**

Standing with your feet shoulder-width apart, interlock your fingers and stretch them over your head with the palms facing toward the ceiling (Figure 13.3). Hold the stretch for 20 seconds. Instead of interlocking your fingers, you can modify this stretch by holding a long pole such as a broomstick over your head and stretching it toward the ceiling.

Bring your right arm across your body. Use your left hand to hold your upper right arm and help pull it across your body (Figure 13.4). Hold for 20 seconds and then repeat with the opposite arm. Repeat 3 times.

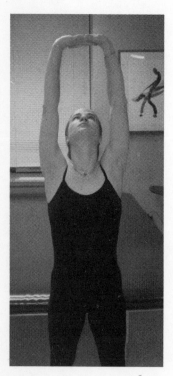

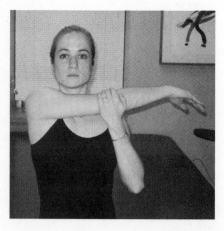

LEFT: 13.3
BELOW: 13.4

Standing with your feet shoulder-width apart, hold a towel with your right arm above and behind your head so that it drops down your back. With your left arm, reach behind your back (around your waist) and grab the dangling towel. With your right arm, pull upward so that your left arm is stretched (Figure 13.5A). Hold for 20 seconds. Then, allow your left arm to pull on the towel to stretch your right arm (Figure 13.5B). Hold for 20 seconds. Repeat using the opposite arms. Do this exercise only once if you have already done the other two shoulder stretching exercises.

13.5A

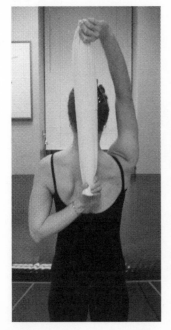

13.5B

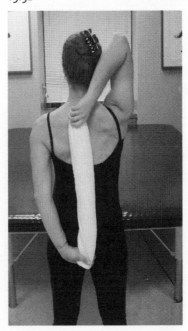

▶ **Chest:**

With your feet shoulder-width apart, hold a long pole over your head with both hands. You may use a broomstick for this purpose or purchase an exercise bar. Slowly lower the pole behind your head until you feel the stretch or the pole come to rest at the base of your neck (Figure 13.6). Hold this pose for 10–20 seconds. Do this only once.

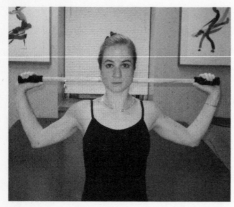

13.6

Hold your arm raised to the side to 90 degrees with the elbow flexed to 90 degrees. Stand next to a wall and place your elbow and forearm against it. Twist gently away from the wall while keeping your forearm and elbow against it so that you stretch your front chest (Figure 13.7). Hold for 10 seconds. Repeat this on the other side of your body. Hold for 10 seconds. Repeat 3 times.

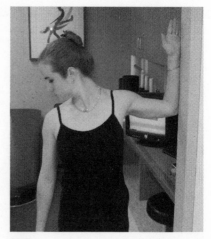

13.7

▶ **Wrist and Hands:**

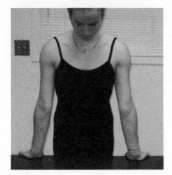

13.8

Stand in front of a table and place your hands on it, palms down so that your fingers are spread out in a fan position, flat on the table. In this position, your fingers should be closer to your body than your palms. If you don't feel the stretch in this position, slowly lean backward until you feel the stretch—but not pain—in your forearms, wrist, and fingers (Figure 13.8). Hold for 30 seconds.

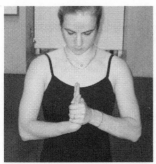

13.9

With your left hand, grab the outside of your right thumb and gently twist your wrist, using your thumb as a fulcrum, so that your right pinky is closest to your chest. (Figure 13.9) Hold this position for 10 seconds. Repeat on the other side of your body. Hold for 10 seconds. Repeat 3 times

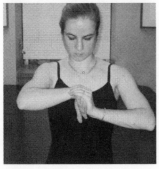

13.10

Hold both arms outstretched in front of you. Turn your right hand so that your right palm faces the same direction as your left. Now bring both hands to your chest (Figure 13.10). Hold for 5 seconds. Repeat on the other side of your body. Hold for 5 seconds. Repeat 2 times.

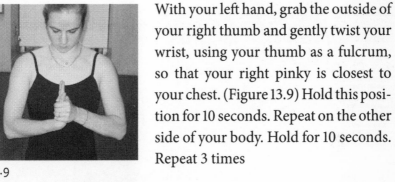

▶ **Mid and Lower Back:**

Lie on an exercise mat face down with your arms on the mat palms down (Figure 13.11A). Slowly raise your head and upper chest off the mat. Walk your hands up so that you are resting on your elbows (Figure 13.11B). Hold the pose for 30 seconds. If you have lower back pain, do not do this exercise unless directed by a physician, as it may worsen your pain.

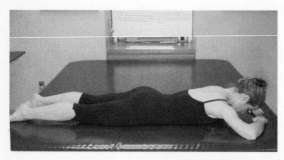

LEFT: 13.11A
BELOW: 13.11B

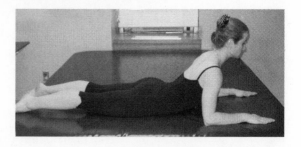

This is an excellent stretch for your lower back if your knees will tolerate it. Lie on your back with your knees bent and your feet flat on the floor. Grab your right knee and gently pull it to your chest so that it points to your right shoulder (Figure 13.12A). Pull your knee to your shoulder as far as it can go without pain. Hold for 10 seconds and then allow your right foot to return to the floor. Repeat this on your left side. Hold for 10 seconds. Now bring both knees to your chest, angling them both so that they point to the shoulder on the same side (Figure 13.12B). Hold for 10 seconds. Repeat this entire procedure 2 times.

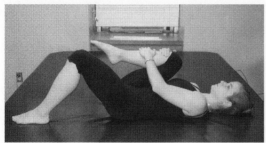

LEFT: 13.12A

BELOW: 13.12B

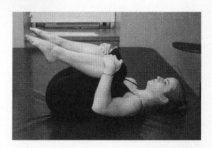

## Legs

▶ **Hamstring stretch:**

Stand with your legs shoulder-width apart and bend forward slowly, keeping your entire back and knees straight, and bending only from your hips. Reach out for the ground with your palms down, trying to touch the floor (Figure 13.13). Feel the stretch in the back of your thighs. Take it very slowly at first, and remember to feel the stretch but don't cause pain. (Don't sacrifice form for increased "motion.") If you bend from your lower back or bend your knees, you will certainly be

13.13

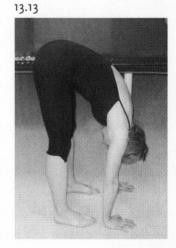

able to reach lower. However, the purpose of this exercise is to stretch the hamstrings in the back of your thighs, not necessarily to actually reach the floor. Bending your knees and/or lower back will only stress these joints and will not help stretch your hamstrings.

Some people, who can't come close to the floor, find it helpful to perform a modified version of this stretch. To do this, place a chair in front of you and reach down for the chair (Figure 13.14). If you can't reach the chair without breaking form, place pillows on the chair until you can reach over and touch the pillows, bending only from the hips. As you become more flexible, you will be able to remove the pillows from the chair. Eventually, you will be able to forgo the chair and reach down to your ankles, and perhaps your feet and even the floor.

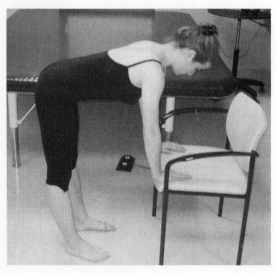

13.14

▶ **Another hamstring stretch:**

Try this hamstring stretch if your lower back hurts. Lie on your back with your legs fully extended. Flatten your back so there is no space between your lumbar spine and the mat. You can do this by contracting your gluteal muscles (also called *glutes* or *buttocks*) to raise them slightly off the mat. You should also contract your abdominal muscles, pushing your belly button into the mat. This is a good strengthening exercise that will help protect your lower back.

Next, bend your left knee so that your left foot is flat on the mat. Now, lift your right leg up to the ceiling, keeping your leg completely straight and your ankle bent. Lift your leg as far as it will go (Figure 13.15). If your hamstrings are relatively flexible, you may be able to get your right leg to 90 degrees. If not, don't be discouraged. Your goal is to increase your flexibility, slowly and smoothly. Hold this stretch for 20 seconds. Remember to keep your back flat on the mat by contracting your gluteal and abdominal muscles. Return to the starting position. Repeat this exercise with

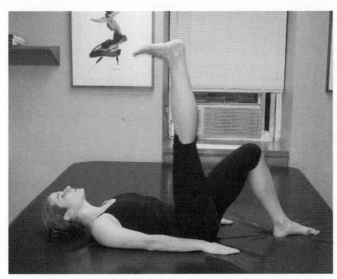

13.15

the other leg. Hold for 20 seconds. Repeat this entire procedure 3 times. This exercise stretches the hamstrings, and it also stretches the calf muscles and strengthens the hip flexors, gluteal muscles, and abdominal muscles.

▶ **Quadriceps stretch:**

Stand in front of a chair or wall. With your left hand, support yourself using the wall or chair. Bend your right knee and grab your right ankle with your right hand behind you. Pull your right ankle backward so that you feel a stretch in the front of your right thigh. Don't pull your right ankle directly up to your right buttock. Instead, concentrate on pulling it up toward the ceiling and backward away from your buttocks (Figure 13.16). This way you won't compress your right knee too much and overstress the cartilage and other structures in your knee. If this pose is difficult, an alternate method is to place a chair behind you and bend your right knee

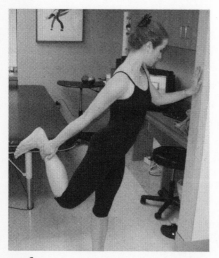

13.16

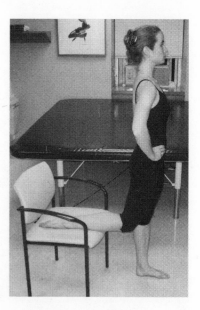

13.17

so that your right shin rests on the chair (Figure 13.17). (You can place a pillow or cushion on the chair for comfort.) The point is to feel the stretch in the front of your left thigh. Hold for 20 seconds. Repeat on the other side. Hold for 20 seconds. Repeat the entire procedure 2 times.

## ▶ Hip flexor stretch:

The hip flexors are also in the front of your thigh, but they are a bit higher up than the quadriceps. The quadriceps stretch will partially stretch these muscles. Another good way to stretch them—and that will also stretch the quadriceps—is to kneel on both knees. Now, bend your right leg in front of you with the knee flexed to 90 degrees. Don't let your right knee bend forward past the toes of your right foot as you flex the knee. Contract your abdominal muscles so that you keep your torso upright and straight (Figure 13.18). Feel the stretch in your left hip flexors. If you don't feel the stretch, you can slide your right foot out further in front of you so that you have to lean further into it. Your right knee should continue to be flexed at 90 degrees. The stretch should be in your left hip flexor. Hold the pose for 20 seconds. Repeat on the other side. Hold for 20 seconds. Repeat the entire procedure 3 times.

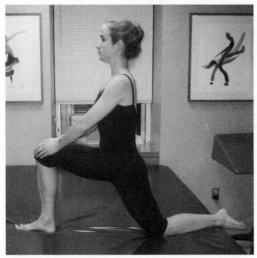

13.18

▶ **Piriformis stretch:**

The piriformis is one of the muscles in the hip area, and it is common for it to become tight. Lie on your back with both knees bent to 90 degrees. Place your right foot in front of your left knee so that it comes to rest on the knee. Next, gently pull your left thigh toward your chest, feeling the stretch in the back of your right buttock (Figure 13.19). This may be an awkward position to get into at first, but it is a wonderful stretch, once you understand how to do it. Remember, stretching should not be painful, so stop if it is. However, try to go slowly, and gently move until you feel the stretch in the back of your buttock. Hold the pose for 20 seconds. Repeat on the other side. Hold for 20 seconds. Repeat the entire procedure 3 times.

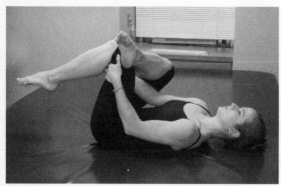

13.19

▶ **Calf and Achilles tendon stretch:**

Stand facing the wall. Place both hands on the wall, with your left leg directly behind the right. Bend your right leg while keeping your left leg completely straight. Lean into the wall and push your left heel into the ground, feeling the stretch in the back of your left calf (Figure 13.20). As you do this, try to bring your toes up off the ground. If you do not feel the stretch, take a few steps back away from the wall and then lean in, repeating the above steps. Hold for 10–20 seconds. Repeat on the other side. Hold for 10–20 seconds. Repeat the entire procedure 3 times.

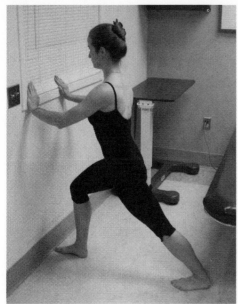

13.20

▶ **Another calf and Achilles tendon stretch:**

This stretch is identical to the previous one, except that the knee is bent while you are stretching your calf and Achilles tendon. By keeping the knee bent, you will stretch a different muscle in your calf. As before, stand facing the wall. Place both hands on the wall, with your left leg directly behind the right. Bend your right leg, this time while keeping your right knee bent at a 30–45 degree angle. Lean into the wall and push your left heel into the ground, feeling the stretch in the back of your left calf. As you do this, try to bring your toes off the ground. If you do not feel the stretch, take a few steps back away from the wall and then lean in, repeating the above steps. Hold for 10–20 seconds. Repeat on the other side. Hold for 10–20 seconds. Repeat the entire procedure 3 times.

# 14

# Principles of Strength Training

ANYONE CAN benefit from strength training, and everyone, to some extent, should include it in her exercise routine. When done in conjunction with stretching and aerobic exercise, it will improve your mobility, decrease pain, and help prevent worsening of arthritis symptoms. The kind of strength training you should do to treat and prevent arthritis is somewhat different than the kind that adds muscle bulk.

How does strength training help? Arthritis involves the loss of some of the cushioning effects of cartilage in a joint. The joint may be painful, swollen, and need protection. Strong, flexible muscles help protect the joints. By being well-toned, the muscles that surround a joint provide a buffer, so the ligaments, bones, and joint capsule don't have to absorb all of the forces acting on it.

## STRENGTH TRAINING BASICS

We have come a long way in our thinking about strength training since the days of Milo, a man from Croton, one of the Greek colonies in Italy. "Milo of Croton" was renowned for his remarkable strength. Legend says he carried a pet calf daily on his back, and continued to carry the animal as it grew into a full-sized ox, thus increasing his strength gradually. Today, as in the time of Milo, strength training involves a gradual increase in weight loading.

Many of the same basic principles that apply to strength training also apply to stretching. The exercises should be performed in a smooth, controlled, deliberate manner. Maintaining good form throughout the exercise is essential to getting the most out of the exercise and avoiding injury.

## Weight-Lifting Terminology

Strength training can be done using weights, so let's briefly cover some weight-lifting terminology. A single movement through a given exercise is called a *repetition*. For example, holding a dumbbell in your hand and doing a bicep curl—flexing your elbow so you raise the dumbbell toward your shoulder, then pausing and lowering it to return to the starting position—is a repetition. A *set* is a series of repetitions performed without taking a break. In general, each set should consist of 10–12 repetitions.

Finally, each repetition has a *positive* and *negative* phase. The positive phase of the repetition is when the muscle is contracting. In the biceps curl, the positive phase is when you are raising the weight against gravity. During this motion, the biceps muscle contracts, becoming shorter. The negative phase of the repetition is when the muscle elongates (lengthens). In the biceps curl, the negative phase is when you lower the weight and straighten your arm.

It is more difficult to perform the negative phase of a repetition than the positive one. Weight lifters who want to grow bigger, stronger muscles often concentrate on the negative phase of their repetitions. Doing this causes more of what is termed "muscle damage." It is actually good to cause muscle damage while lifting weights, because it is not really damage. Rather, it is the process of breaking down weaker muscle so you can build bigger, stronger muscle.

## DON'T STOP BREATHING!

Blood pressure increases during weight training, especially during the negative phase of a repetition. You should never hold your breath while lifting weights, which can lead to dangerously high blood pressure. Exhale during the negative phase; and inhale during the positive phase.

We will discuss specific strength training exercises later in this chapter, but remember that everyone is different and that a personalized exercise plan developed by a qualified physician can be of great benefit. However, the general routine that most people follow is: 1–3 exercises per muscle group, 2–5 sets per exercise, and 6–12 repetitions per set.

## TYPES OF MUSCLES

There are two important types of skeletal muscle. *Type I*, also called *slow-twitch*, is composed of small fibers and is used primarily for carrying light loads. This type of fiber predominates in a runner who is very thin and whose body contains a lot of lean muscle. A marathon runner's leg muscles contain an abundance of well-exercised type I muscle fibers.

*Type II* muscle fibers, also called *fast-twitch*, are large muscle fibers used for lifting heavy loads. A weight lifter has an abundance of type II muscle fibers. Competitive sprinters also have plenty of type II muscle fibers in their large leg muscles, which are used to produce strong movements for a short time.

In general, lifting a heavier weight for 2–8 repetitions per set primarily exercises your type II muscle fibers, and will produce large muscles capable of lifting heavier loads for short periods of time. If you lift a lighter weight for 8–15 repetitions, you are exercising primarily your type I muscle fibers. This type of exercise will result in smaller, leaner muscles that are capable of lifting light loads for longer periods of time. If you lift a very light weight for more than 20 repetitions, you are really doing aerobic exercise rather than strength training. If you are trying to build strength, the weight needs to be heavier than you can comfortably use for 20 repetitions.

In order to treat and prevent arthritis, you should exercise a combination of type I and II muscles, with a slight emphasis on the type I slow-twitch fibers. Aim to complete 8–12 repetitions for each set. You should perform 3–5 sets per muscle exercise, and do 1–3 exercises per muscle group. You should increase the weight once you can perform 12 repetitions for 3 sets with only mild fatigue.

## A Word about Repetitions

Form is foremost. Think about your form not just for the muscle you are exercising, but for your entire body. For example, if you are doing a standing biceps curl, it is important that you focus on your biceps, elbow, hand, wrist, and shoulder. It is also important to maintain good body posture while doing the curl, with your feet shoulder-width apart, abdominal muscles slightly contracted to protect your spine, feet flat on the ground, and knees minimally flexed (about 3–4 degrees). We'll talk about form in greater detail when we discuss specific exercises. For now, just appreciate that, when exercising, it is important to be aware of your entire body posture in addition to the muscle being exercised.

The positive phase of contracting the muscle should last 2 seconds. Pause at the end of the contraction for less than 1 second and then lower the weight into the negative phase of the repetition for 3 seconds. A full repetition should last no less than 5 seconds.

Remember to inhale during the positive phase and exhale during the negative phase.

Time the phases by counting out loud. At the very least, you will need to count in your head when you first start to exercise, but I recommend counting out loud until it becomes automatic. Don't cheat yourself by doing a quicker, easier repetition. Take a breath, 2 seconds up while inhaling, pause, and 3 seconds down while exhaling. Repeat. Work your muscles, and your joints will thank you.

# 15.

## Strength Training Exercises

THERE IS no substitute for learning directly from someone with experience and knowledge. It is a mistake to learn how to exercise only from a book or video, even this one! As stated several times previously, always exercise under the direct guidance of a qualified trainer. You will need to ask the trainer questions, at least in the beginning. For example, you might ask, "Am I doing this right?" Show the trainer how you perform the exercise, and work on improving your form or changing the exercise to something that will produce better results.

Every person's body responds differently to different exercises, and your training needs will change as your body begins to respond to different exercises and your muscles develop. Strength training is an evolving process that works best when you have a qualified coach. Muscles get used to certain exercises, and you have to surprise them with different, new exercises if you want them to respond optimally.

A good book on strength training exercises should give you the information you need to open a meaningful dialogue with your physician, physical therapist, and/or trainer. By having a basic understanding of the principles involved in strength training and some core exercises, you can engage your doctor and/or trainer much more easily in a discussion of what exercises are right for you.

## NECESSARY PRECAUTIONS

If you develop chest pain, headache, nausea, vomiting, dizziness, or have prolonged difficulty catching your breath while exercising, stop and contact your doctor immediately.

In addition to any heart, lung, or other systemic problems that might preclude your participation in an exercise regimen, there are other reasons why you may need to forgo or modify some exercises, particularly strength training exercises. For example, if you have a shoulder problem, such as impingement syndrome or a rotator cuff tear, you may not be able to do certain chest and shoulder exercises, and may have to forgo any over-the-head strength training until the condition improves. If you have a pinched nerve in your back, certain core strengthening exercises would be contraindicated.

Strength training may cause a burning sensation in the muscles you are exercising. This is normal. However, stop exercising if you experience excessive pain. If you have a known musculoskeletal problem, such as hip labral tear, rotator cuff tendonitis, or discogenic back pain, talk to your doctor and physical therapist before beginning an exercise program to find out which exercises are safe for you. Sometimes, you might only need to modify an existing exercise.

As with the stretches, I did not invent these exercises. After reviewing hundreds of exercises, I have found these to be the best starting point for my patients and for me. When necessary, I have modified them from their usual form. I have included enough exercises in areas such as core strengthening so you can pick and choose those that are the most comfortable for you. If you have time, consider doing all of them. If you are pressed for time, alternate core strengthening exercises to keep your workout interesting, both for you and for your muscles.

## Thigh Muscles

▶ **The squat:**

This is a wonderful exercise for the quadriceps, hamstrings, and buttocks. If you can only do one exercise for your lower extremities, this would probably be the one. Stand with a chair behind you (or possibly without a chair once you are comfortable with the exercise), with your feet shoulder-width apart and firmly planted on the ground. At no time during this exercise should your feet leave the ground or should you elevate onto your toes. Your back should remain straight, and your abdominal muscles must remain contracted to help protect your lower back. Slowly bend your knees as if you were going to sit on the chair. Drop your buttocks straight backward and raise your arms up and forward to help with control and balance (Figure 15.1). Don't let your knees come forward past your toes. As you lower yourself, raise your arms up straight in front of you.

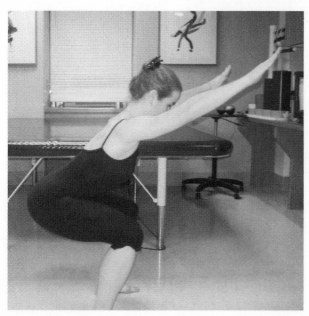

15.1

▶ **Modified squat:**

Alternatively, simply cross your arms across your chest so that your right hand holds your left shoulder and your left hand holds your right shoulder. As you lower yourself toward the chair, remember to exhale (Figure 15.2). Before sitting in the chair, pause so that your thighs are parallel with the ground. Then, slowly stand up, keeping your abdominal muscles contracted and your back straight. This is one repetition of a true squat, but we call it a *modified squat* because if you find it too difficult, you can place pillows on the chair. In this way, you lower yourself only to the pillows so that your thighs never become parallel with the floor. Start with as many pillows as you need. As you improve and become familiar with the mechanics of the exercise, you will need fewer and fewer pillows. Eventually, you should be able to get your thighs parallel (or close to parallel) with the floor. Again, the purpose of the exercise is not to "get parallel" but rather to strengthen your leg muscles.

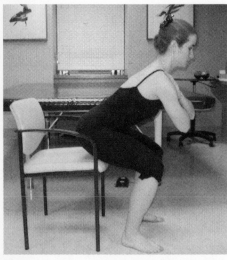

15.2

Never sacrifice form to be able to lower yourself more. This exercise might feel awkward at first, but it will soon become easier. A doctor, physical therapist, or qualified trainer will be invaluable in helping you to perfect your form. Once you can do 4 sets of 12 repetitions without too much difficulty, you can progress to carrying 5–10 pound weights (or heavier) in your hands at your sides while doing the exercise. But first, perfect the exercise without any weight.

▶ **Front of the thigh:**

Sit in a chair with your feet dangling, but not touching the floor. You may need to use a pillow on the seat to lift yourself slightly higher. Make sure you are secure in your seat so you won't fall off. Grip the sides of the chair for support (Figure 15.3A). With your feet pointing only slightly outward to the sides, slowly extend your left leg (Figure 15.3B). Remember to exhale as you do this. Don't lock your knee. Extend it so that it is almost completely straight, but not quite. Pause and slowly flex your knee so it returns to the starting position. Next, do the same with your right knee. Perform three sets. If you find this exercise easy, attach a 2-pound ankle weight (which you can purchase at any exercise equipment store). Increase the weight when you can do 3 sets of 12 repetitions.

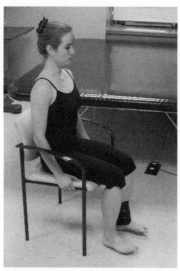
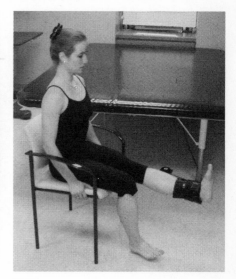

15.3A          15.3B

▶ **Strengthening the hamstrings:**

Lie face down on a padded exercise bench so that your legs dangle off the side and you can hold onto the ends of the bench for support. Your bed can serve this purpose if you don't have a bench at home. Lie face down, across the width of the bed, allowing your knees and lower legs to dangle over the side. Reach your arms in front of you and grab the opposite side of the bed for support. Slowly flex your right knee until it is at a 90-degree angle (Figure 15.4). Pause, and

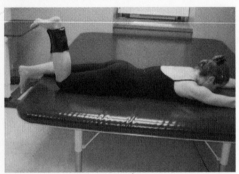

then extend your knee so it returns to being parallel with the floor. Repeat with your left leg. If this exercise is easy to perform for 3 sets of 12 repetitions each, use an ankle weight. This exercise is good for strengthening

15.4

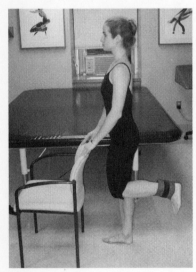

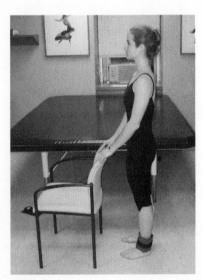

15.5A                              15.5A

your hamstrings. Alternatively, simply stand in front of a chair or the wall (Figure 15.5A). Hold onto it for support and flex your left knee until it comes to 90 degrees (Figure 15.5B). Pause, and then slowly extend the knee so that your foot returns to the floor. Remember to use good breathing technique. Repeat with your right leg. If you have lower back pain, the standing hamstring strengthening exercise will be best for you. You may need ankle weights to add resistance for this alternate exercise if you can perform 3 sets of 12 repetitions.

## HIPS

▶ **Back of the hip:**

Lie on an exercise mat with your stomach on the mat. You may use one pillow to rest your head on and another to support your pelvis (Figure 15.6A). Keeping your legs straight, raise your right leg off the mat (Figure 15.6B). Feel the squeeze in your buttocks. Pause, then slowly lower your leg to the mat. Repeat with your left leg. As

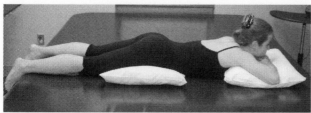

15.6A

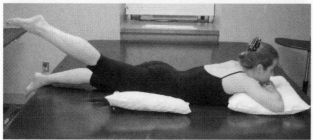

15.6B

you improve, you may need to use ankle weights to increase resistance. Placing a pillow beneath your pelvis can make this exercise more comfortable. Perform 3 sets of 12 repetitions on both sides.

▶ **Outside of the hip:**

Lie on the exercise mat on your left side. Bend your left knee so that your foot is behind you. Keep your right leg straight (Figure 15.7A). Slowly raise your right leg up in the air, so that it makes about a 45-degree angle with your body (Figure 15.7B). Feel the squeeze in the outside of your hip. Pause, and allow your leg to align with your body. If possible, do not allow your right leg to lower all the way to the floor (Figure 15.7C). Instead, pause when it aligns with

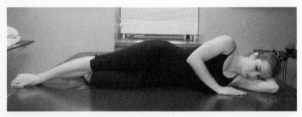

15.7A

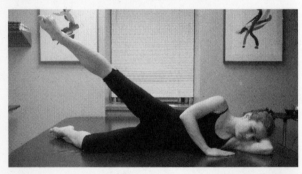

15.7B

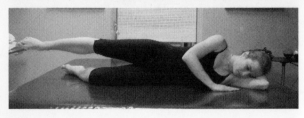

15.7C

your body, and then raise it again to 45 degrees. Repeat this for 8–12 repetitions. If you can't stop your leg when it aligns with your body, allow it to slowly lower to the ground and then repeat. Turn onto your right side and repeat the exercise with your left leg. Once you can do 3 sets of 12 repetitions, add 2-pound ankle weights.

▶ **Inner thigh:**

A good way to exercise the inside of your thighs is to lie on your back with your feet straight up in the air so that your hips are bent at approximately 90 degrees. It is okay if you need to bend your knees a bit (Figure 15.8A). Allow your legs to slowly fall to the sides so that they make a "V" in the air. Pause when you feel a slight stretch

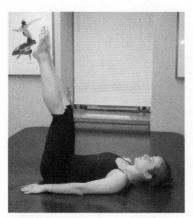
15.8A

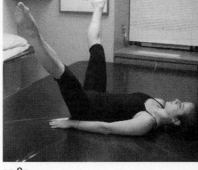
15.8B

in your inner thighs—this should occur when your thighs form approximately a 60–90 degree angle, depending on your flexibility (Figure 15.8B). After a brief pause, squeeze your thighs together to bring your legs back to midline. Pause and repeat. Do 3 sets of 12 repetitions. If your back hurts while doing this exercise, try doing a posterior pelvic tilt at the same time (see core strengthening for details on how to do this). If your pain persists, try using your hands to support your buttocks. If pain persists despite these modifications, stop the exercise.

▶ **Calves:**

Stand on a stair with your toes or balls of your feet on the edge of the step, with the middle of your feet and heels hanging off the edge. Hold on to a sturdy railing or wall for support (Figure 15.9A). Push down with your toes so that you raise yourself up and are standing on your tip-toes (Figure 15.9B). Pause and then slowly lower

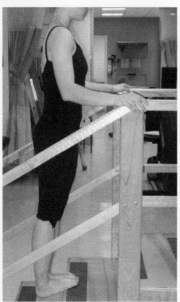

15.9A                          15.9B

yourself down so that your heels lower down beneath the step. You should feel a very slight stretch in the back of your calves. If you feel more than a slight stretch, your calves are probably tight. Pause with your heels down, then rise up again to stand on your tip-toes. Your feet should be shoulder-width apart. Your back should be straight and your stomach slightly contracted. Remember to exhale as you rise up on your toes and slowly inhale as you slowly lower yourself so that your heels are down. If this exercise becomes too easy, you can try doing it one foot at a time, but remember to hold onto the railing or wall for support. If this becomes too easy, you can hold a small weight with one hand and the railing or wall with the other. Perform 3 sets of 12 repetitions. Note that the model in Figure 15 is using a piece of equipment for the exercise. This is one of the advantages of being in a gym or physical therapy setting. However, you don't need a piece of equipment like this to perform the exercise. You just need to be in a place that has steps and a secure banister or wall for you to hold onto so you don't lose your balance.

## CORE STRENGTHENING

▶ **Posterior pelvic tilt:**

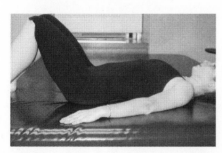

15.10A

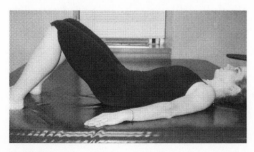

15.10B

This is perhaps the best and safest way for many people to exercise their abdominal muscles.

Start by lying on your back on an exercise mat or carpet. Bend your knees so your feet are flat on the mat (Figure 15.10A). Squeeze your gluteal muscles together so they rise slightly off the mat. At the same time, contract your abdominal muscles. The curve in your lumbar spine should straighten, and your lower back should be flat against the mat (Figure 15.10B). If you are not sure, check your position by trying to place your hand underneath your lower back. In this position, you should not be able to do this. Next, bring both knees to your chest. Then straighten your right leg while keeping your left knee at your chest with about 90-degree flexion in the hip (Figure 15.10C). Next, bend your right leg so that your right knee comes

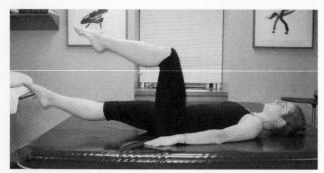

15.10C

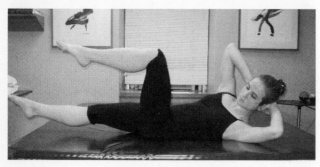

15.10D

to your chest, and then straighten your left leg. It is as if you are lying on the ground and riding a bicycle in midair with your gluteal and abdominal muscles contracted to reverse the lumbar curve and protect your back. This is a challenging activity. At first, you might only be able to straighten your lumbar curve. After you can straighten your lumbar curve easily, begin to bend and straighten your legs. When you can do 3 sets of 12 repetitions while bending and straightening your legs, you can begin to bring your arms into the exercise. Do this by folding your arms behind your head. As you bring your right knee to your chest, move your left elbow toward the right knee. Then repeat with your left knee and right elbow (Figure 15.10D). Most importantly, continue to squeeze your gluteal and abdominal muscles so that your back remains flat on the mat, reversing the lumbar curve. As always, do not sacrifice your form. The form in this exercise requires particularly attention to detail, and physician or trainer instruction and guidance is strongly recommended.

A good strength training exercise for your back is to lie face down on the exercise mat with your arms at your sides, thumbs close to your body, palms up. Slowly lift your head and chest up off the mat about 4–6 inches, or until it is no longer comfortable (Figure 15.11A). Keep your spine in alignment by keeping your neck, chest, and back straight. Pause, and then return to rest your chest for less than a second on the mat. Then repeat. This can be a difficult exer-

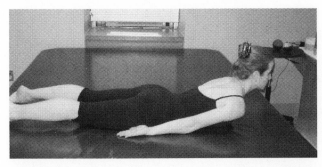

15.11A

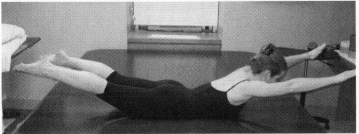

15.11B

cise. If you experience any pain stop the exercise. Although most people can do this exercise, some back conditions can be worsened by it, so be cautious. If you master the exercise, a more advanced form is to raise your legs and arms off the mat at the same time and hold the pose (Figure 15.11B).

▶ **Core strengthening with the "bridge":**

With your knees bent at a 90-degree angle and your feet flat on the ground, contract your gluteal and abdominal muscles and raise your abdomen and buttocks off the ground so that your body is straight from your chest to your knees (Figure 15.12). This is an excellent exercise for your core muscles as well as your glutes. Concentrate on keeping your abdominals and gluteal muscles contracted and tight at all times during the exercise. It may help to think of driving your heels into the ground. (Some people call this a *bridge*). Hold this position for 10 seconds. Repeat 3 times.

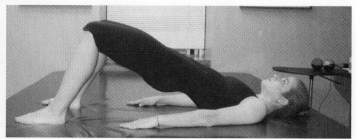

15.12

A good abdominal exercise is to lie with your back flat on the ground and knees and hips bent at approximately 90 degrees (Figure 15.13A). Slowly, in a controlled manner, with your abdominals contracted, tap your right toes on the mat. Keep your knees bent at 90 degrees at all times. Only extend your hip, one at a time, so that you can tap the mat with your foot (Figure 15.13B). Once you have tapped the mat with your right toes, bring your right hip back to 90 degrees and then tap the mat with your left toes. Each time you have touched the mat with your right and left toes (in succession), you have completed one repetition. Do 3 sets of 15 repetitions. If you experience pain while doing this exercise, you can perform a posterior pelvic tilt at the same time. If the pain persists, discontinue the exercise and discuss it with your doctor, physical therapist, or trainer.

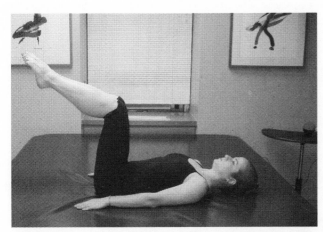

15.13A

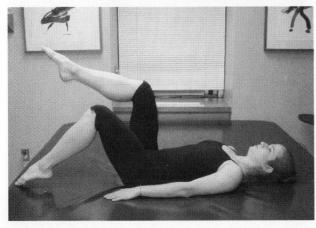

15.13B

## ADVANCED CORE STRENGTHENING

This is another terrific, though somewhat challenging, exercise for your back and entire body: Kneel on all fours with your back straight (Figure 15.14A). Simultaneously extend your left arm and right leg out straight so that your arm reaches forward as far as possible and your leg extends back (Figure 15.14B). Some people call this the *quadruped* exercise. Hold the pose for 10–15 seconds. Repeat using the opposite leg and arm. Repeat the entire exercise 3 times. If lifting the leg and opposite arm at the same time is too difficult at first, an alternative is to lift one arm, return to neutral, and then lift the opposite leg. Then repeat with the other limbs.

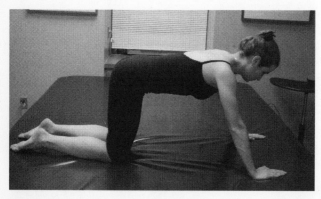

LEFT: 15.14A

BELOW: 15.14B

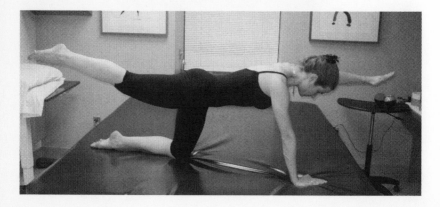

Another good exercise is to lie on your stomach, keeping your back straight and abdominal muscles contracted. Support yourself on your elbows (with your palms face down) and toes (Figure 15.15). This is commonly called a *modified plank* position. Hold the position for 15–20 seconds. Rest for a few seconds. Repeat 3 times.

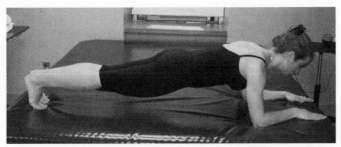

15.15

A more advanced exercise is to lie on your side and lift yourself up on your elbow. Keep your body straight. While lying on your left side, lift your right hip up into the air. Hold the position and raise your right arm into the air, extending it up to the ceiling (Figure 15.16). Some people like to look up at their extended hand as they

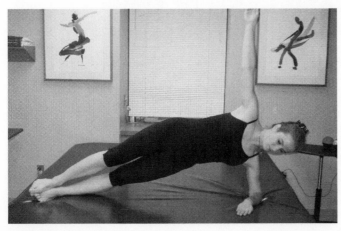

15.16

perform this *modified side plank* exercise. Hold this position for 10 seconds. Repeat on the other side. Repeat the entire exercise 3 times.

## CHEST AND TRICEPS

Push-ups are a great way to exercise your upper body. A full push-up involves supporting yourself with your hands and toes. Contract your abdominal muscles. Keep your back perfectly straight (Figure 15.17A). Slowly lower yourself by bending your elbows until your nose and chest almost touch the ground (Figure 15.17B). Pause and then push up so that you raise your trunk until your arms are fully extended. Be sure to keep your back perfectly straight throughout the entire exercise. Doing this in front of a mirror to monitor your posture helps.

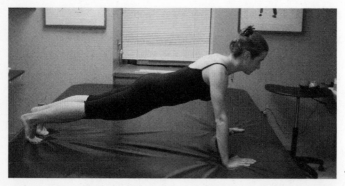

15.17A

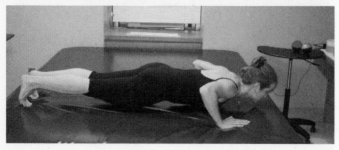

15.17B

Doing 10 proper push-ups is difficult for many people. If you have trouble doing more than 4 (many if not most people who don't regularly exercise do have trouble with this), I recommend starting the exercise with your knees (instead of your toes) on the ground. Keep your back perfectly straight and your abdominal muscles contracted as you perform the exercise (Figure 15.18A). Slowly lower yourself by bending your elbows, until your nose and chest almost touch the ground (Figure 15.18B).

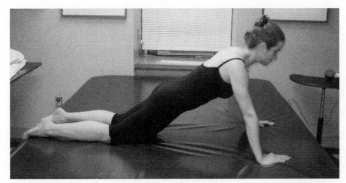

15.18A

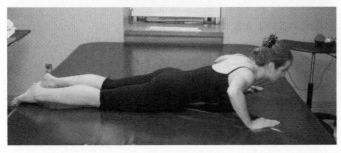

15.18B

An alternative to this is to bend your knees and cross your legs as you do the modified push-up on the ground (Figure 15.19A,B). If this is also too difficult, try a standing push-up. Stand in front of the wall with your arms extended and hands on the wall (Figure 15.20A). Slowly lean into the wall, supporting yourself with your

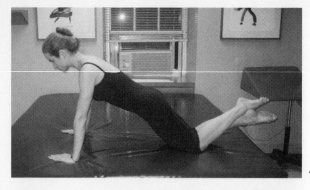

15.19A

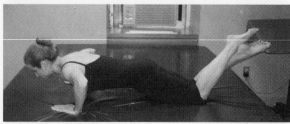

LEFT:15.19B

BELOW:
LEFT: 15.20A
RIGHT: 15.20B

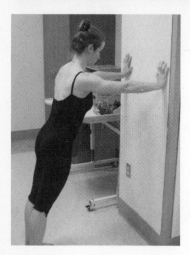

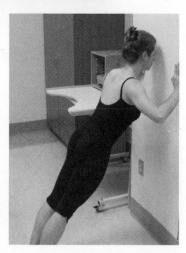

hands (Figure 15.20B). Push against the wall to return to the fully upright position. Once you can do three sets of 12 repetitions, proceed to the push-ups with your knees on the ground. Once you can do those, proceed to the full push-ups. You can try doing your first set of push-ups with your knees on the ground. Then, for the second and third sets, you can go to standing push-ups.

## SHOULDERS

Sitting in a chair, hold a 3-pound dumbbell in each hand (these can be purchased from a sporting good store if you are exercising at home). Your hands should hang at your sides. Turn your hands so that your thumbs face 45 degrees to the outside (Figure 15.21A). This is important particularly if you have ever had any shoulder pain because, by rotating your thumbs outward, you actually also rotate part of the bone in your shoulder so that it does not rub against the tendons that often causes shoulder pain. If you have had shoulder pain, or have been told you have impingement syndrome, try keeping your thumbs pointing up whenever you are carrying anything, including weights or groceries. With the weights at your side, raise your arms out to your sides as if you were

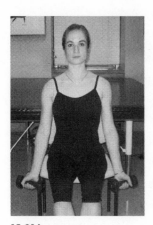
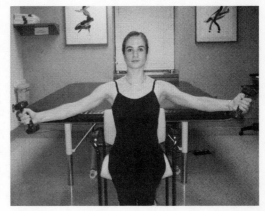

15.21A                    15.21B

trying to fly (Figure 15.21B). Be sure to keep your arms slightly bent at the elbows to keep pressure off of these joints. Do not swing your arms; keep the movement slow and controlled. Don't bend your wrists, but keep them in an even line with your arm. As you raise the weights, remember to inhale and keep your stomach muscles contracted to protect your spine. Pause when your arms are at 90 degrees to your body (level with your shoulders) and slowly lower the weights as you exhale. Repeat. Once you can do 3 sets of 12 repetitions, increase the weight. Alternatively, you can do this exercise while standing. If you choose to stand, be sure to keep your knees slightly bent (3–5 degrees), your abdominal muscles contracted, and your back straight.

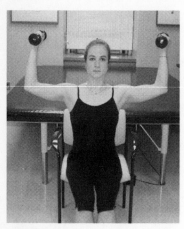

15.22A

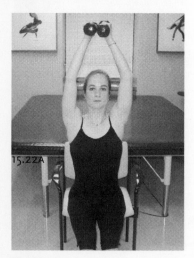

15.22A

15.22B

Still sitting in the chair holding the 3-pound dumbbells, hold your arms up at your sides as if you were showing off your biceps (Figure 15.22A). Next, with your palms facing inward to your body, raise the dumbbells over your head and bring them together as you straighten your elbows (Figure 15.22B). Feel the contraction in your shoulders. Pause at the top of the motion, then bring the dumbbells down to your sides. Be sure to keep your back straight and your stomach muscles contracted throughout this movement. If you need to arch your back to get the weight above your head, use a lighter weight. Keep your abdominal muscles contracted throughout the movement. Remember to inhale as you extend your arms over your head, and exhale as you bring your arms down until your elbows are at 90 degrees. Do not drop your elbows beneath your shoulders. Once you can do 3 sets of 12 repetitions, increase the weight.

## BICEPS

The best way to perform the biceps curl is in the seated position. Keep your back straight and your stomach muscles slightly contracted. Hold two dumbbells at your sides. Use a small amount of weight until you can perform three sets of 12 repetitions with

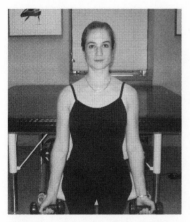

15.23A

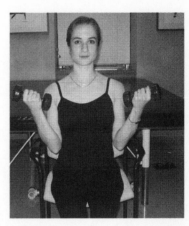

15.23B

good form. Your palms should face outward so that your little fingers are closest to your body (Figure 15.23A). As you bring the weight up, bending only at your elbows, turn your little fingers outward at the top of the repetition (Figure 15.23B). Pause at the very top of the contraction, then slowly return to the starting position. Remember to keep your elbows close to your body, with no visible space in between. Alternatively, you can do this exercise while standing. If you choose to stand, be sure to keep your knees slightly bent (3–5 degrees), your abdominal muscles contracted, and your back straight.

## Triceps

While seated and maintaining good trunk posture, raise your right hand over your head. Use a small weight initially for this exercise. Keeping your right arm above your head next to your ear, flex your right elbow to 90 degrees so that your hand drops behind your head (Figure 15.24A). Inhale as you do this, and exhale as you straighten your arm (Figure 15.24B). Do 12 repetitions, then repeat with your

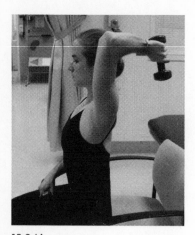

15.24A

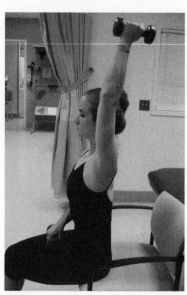

15.24B

left arm. Increase the weight once you can do 3 sets. Alternatively, you can do this exercise while standing. If you choose to stand, be sure to keep your knees slightly bent (3–5 degrees), your abdominal muscles contracted, and your back straight.

## Forearms, Wrist, and Hands

There are many ways to strengthen your forearms, wrists, and hands. You can use small weights and isolate the muscles. Another good way is to simply use a tension ball and squeeze it periodically while watching television or reading a book. Simply continue to repeat the squeezes and remember to switch hands.

### "No Pain, No Gain" Does Not Apply to Joints!

If you have a painful joint as the result of arthritis, you may need to modify some exercises to avoid overstressing that joint. On the other hand, *do not stop moving a painful joint.* We have already discussed how the joint will lose its nourishment and quickly start to become fibrotic and more painful if you simply stop bending it or using it at all. As it becomes more painful, you will use it even less. This cycle will result in a joint that ultimately may require surgery. You can stop this cycle by learning to exercise the joint in a constructive way.

If you feel pain in a joint while exercising, take a short break. Be sure to emphasize stretching and strengthening the muscles around the painful joint(s), but remember that the entire body is connected, and you should exercise all your muscles for optimal benefit—and also to help protect against developing pain in other joints in the future. It's okay to work through muscle pain, but never through joint pain. If you are unsure whether or not pain is muscular or from the joint, stop and ask your doctor. She may suggest you take a mild over-the-counter pain medication prior to exercise. Always talk to your physician before taking medication, because you don't want to mask increasing joint pain.

# 16.

## Aerobic Exercise

No exercise program would be complete without aerobic exercise. One popular sequence of exercise is a warm-up period followed by aerobic exercise, strengthening exercises, and then stretching. An alternative routine is a warm-up followed by stretching, strengthening, and then aerobic exercise.

There are many ways to get aerobic exercise. You can rake leaves, shovel snow, bicycle, jog, run, walk, swim, play tennis, take an aerobics class, dance, jump rope, roller skate, cross-country ski—the list goes on. It's important to remember that, although weight-bearing activities are important for bone stimulation, bone growth, and the prevention of osteoporosis, many people with arthritis cannot tolerate certain weight-bearing activities. For example, jogging is an excellent aerobic activity, but it may not be a realistic option for someone who has severe arthritis of the knee—at least not until the symptoms are better controlled.

An elliptical machine is ideal for people with arthritis, because it is weight-bearing, but without the impact of jogging or walking. You can comfortably use it in rain, sleet, snow, or excessive heat because it is kept indoors. People tend to stick with activities that they enjoy and that are weather-independent. You can use it in front of a television, while reading a book, or listening to music, which will make it more likely that you will stick with it. Other machines fit these criteria, including stationary bicycles and treadmills (although treadmills are high-impact and can overstress the joints). If you use a stationary bicycle, adjust the pedals so that you don't bring your knees to more than 90 degrees of flexion.

The most important factor in choosing an aerobic exercise is to choose one that you will actually *do* on a regular basis. An exercise regimen of 30 minutes of jogging every day won't do you any good if you hate to jog and quit after two days, or only manage to do it once a week. Do whatever you can to make your workout fun and interesting so you will stick with it. In my experience, for most people, this means doing aerobics in front of the television or while reading a book. Find the exercise that is right for *you*.

## How Much Aerobic Activity Should I Do?

The U.S. Surgeon General, the Centers for Disease Control and Prevention, and the American College of Sports Medicine all recommend that everyone should get a minimum of 30 minutes of moderate-intensity physical activity most days of the week. "Moderate" activity makes you breathe a little harder and your heart beat a little faster, but still allows you to talk comfortably while exercising; this is called the "talk test." The experts recommend that the 30 minutes of activity be done either all at once or divided into 10–15 minute periods.

A minimum of 30 minutes of aerobic activity is a good target, but I believe you should exercise for 30 minutes straight, if possible, rather than breaking it into shorter segments. There is good evidence that cholesterol in the arteries isn't broken down for energy before at least 20 minutes of continuous activity. Therefore, it makes sense that the 30 minutes should be performed at one time for optimal results. Of course, two segments of 15 minutes are better than no exercise at all.

Keep in mind that, as you progress with your exercises, you

will need and want to gradually increase the intensity under the direction of your physician, physical therapist, and/or qualified trainer.

## WAYS TO GET EXTRA AEROBIC EXERCISE

There are many ways to get extra aerobic exercise in addition to your scheduled workouts. Here are some tips:

- Park a little farther from work so you will have to walk more.
- Take a brisk walk during your lunch break.
- Try playing a new sport.
- Walk the golf course instead of using a cart.
- Go dancing.

## THE IMPORTANCE OF COOLING DOWN

Always remember to cool down after exercising. This gives your muscles a chance to relax and prevents your blood pressure from dropping too rapidly, which can happen if your blood is allowed to pool in your extremities.

Exercising activates the *sympathetic nervous system*, the part of the nervous system that is responsible for your body's "flight or fight" response. This is your body's physiologic response to challenges such as running from a saber tooth tiger, defending your home against an intruder, or summoning the nerve to ask someone for a date. Your eyes dilate, heart rate increases, blood pressure rises (in fact, your blood can pump 400–600 percent more than when at rest), and your arteries redirect your blood flow away from your abdomen and to your heart, brain, and extremities (if they are active). When you exercise using your arms and legs, the arteries in your extremities dilate to allow blood to flow to them. When you stop exercising, your sympathetic nervous system turns off and your *parasympathetic nervous system* turns on.

The parasympathetic nervous system takes over when you are at rest, such as immediately after a large meal. Your blood pressure drops, your blood vessels relax and dilate, blood flows to your abdomen, and your heart rate slows. The blood that only moments ago was being powerfully pumped by your sympathetically charged heart no longer has that strong push, and has a tendency to pool in your extremities. The blood does not get to your head, creating the potential for fainting. This can be avoided by cooling down after you exercise.

Ironically, the better the shape you are in, the more you are at risk for fainting post-exercise if you don't have a proper cool down. This is because a person in good shape can make the transition more quickly and efficiently. Have you ever seen runners interviewed after a marathon? What do they do when they cross the finish line? They keep walking. This is the way they cool down, and this is why the interviews after a marathon are "walking interviews." If a marathon runner stopped running immediately and sat down, the blood would pool in her extremities and she might very well faint, not to mention that her muscles would cramp up.

Exercise every day. Make it a routine, part of your daily life. You wouldn't go a day without eating or brushing your teeth, and you should think similarly about exercising. Aerobic activity and stretching should be done at least 5 times per week, and strength training 4 times a week. When you strength-train, exercise different muscles each day; don't exercise the same muscle 2 days in a row. Muscles need at least a day of rest before the next workout. If they don't, you probably aren't working them hard enough. Of course, always remember to use pain as a guide. You may need to build up to more exercise as your pain diminishes.

You are exercising too much if exercising increases your joint swelling, causes pain that lasts for more than 30 minutes after exercising, results in persistent fatigue, or decreases your strength or range of motion. Work with your health care professional to determine the optimal amount of exercise for you.

Other forms of exercise that can be a terrific supplement to your regimen include tai chi or Pilates, which focus on balance, flexibility, and agility. When performed under experienced, expert supervision, yoga can be a wonderful way to decrease stress and improve range of motion, as well as increase strength and cardiovascular ability.

# 17

# Exercise Prescriptions for the Hip and Knee

THIS CHAPTER contains exercise routines tailored to the two parts of the body that are most commonly affected by arthritis: the knee and hip. If your doctor diagnoses arthritis in your knees or hips, these exercises can help. Please read Chapters 13-16 before doing the exercises, and talk to your doctor to make sure they are safe for you.

Exercising the muscles surrounding the knees or hips is helpful if you have arthritis in these joints, but it is better to address the entire body. This chapter takes a more focused approach because many people do not follow through with the more comprehensive program. If this is you, by all means start with these more specific programs, but plan on progressing to a total body workout when you are ready.

## LOWER BACK PAIN

Lower back pain caused by arthritis is a complicated topic. If you have lower back pain, be sure to see a physician who specializes in back pain. Arthritis is only one possible cause for lower back pain, and it is important to have an accurate diagnosis before an exercise prescription can be given, so you will not cause further injury. If you have lower back pain, and have been told by your doctor it is due to arthritis, stretching and strengthening the hip girdle muscles and performing core strengthening exercises should be very helpful. However, if any of these exercises are painful, stop immediately. Do not exercise "through the pain." Talk to your doctor.

## Arthritis of the Knee

Start your workout with a 5–10 minute warm-up, which may be as simple as going for a brisk walk. The point is to get your blood flowing and your heart rate up. Never exercise through joint pain; if your joint hurts, stop and rest, and then gradually ease back into the exercise. If the pain persists, talk to your doctor. You may need to take a mild pain reliever before exercising and ice the painful joint afterwards. Even if the joint is not painful immediately after exercising, ice is a powerful anti-inflammatory. A simple way to ice a joint is to put a bag of frozen peas on the joint for 15–20 minutes. If you have diabetes or any problem with your nerves that make it difficult to feel heat or cold, be careful to not keep the frozen peas (or ice) on for too long, to avoid injuring your skin.

## Begin with These Stretches:

▸ **Hamstring stretch:**

Stand with your legs shoulder-width apart and bend forward slowly, keeping your entire back and knees straight, and bending only from your hips. Reach out for the ground with your palms down, trying to touch the floor (Figure 13.13). Feel the stretch in the back of your thighs. Take it very slowly at first, and remember to feel the stretch but don't cause pain. (Don't sacrifice form for increased "motion.") If you bend from your lower back or bend your knees, you will certainly be able to reach lower. However, the purpose of this exercise is to stretch the hamstrings in the back of your thighs, not necessarily to actually reach the floor. Bending your knees and/or lower back will only stress these joints and will not help stretch your hamstrings.

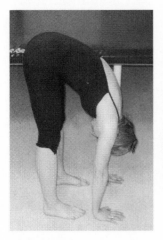
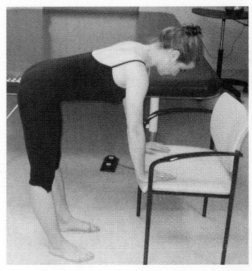

ABOVE: 13.13
RIGHT: 13.14

Some people, who can't come close to the floor, find it helpful to perform a modified version of this stretch. To do this, place a chair in front of you and reach down for the chair (Figure 13.14). If you can't reach the chair without breaking form, place pillows on the chair until you can reach over and touch the pillows, bending only from the hips. As you become more flexible, you will be able to remove the pillows from the chair. Eventually, you will be able to forgo the chair and reach down to your ankles, and perhaps your feet and even the floor.

### ▶ Another hamstring stretch:

Try this hamstring stretch if your lower back hurts. Lie on your back with your legs fully extended. Flatten your back so there is no space between your lumbar spine and the mat. You can do this by contracting your gluteal muscles (also called *glutes* or *buttocks*) to raise them slightly off the mat. You should also contract your abdominal muscles, pushing your belly button into the mat. This is a good strengthening exercise that will help protect your lower back.

Next, bend your left knee so that your left foot is flat on the mat. Now, lift your right leg up to the ceiling, keeping your leg completely straight and your ankle bent. Lift your leg as far as it will go

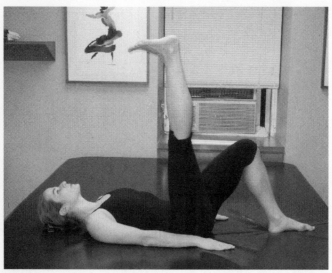

13.15A

(Figure 13.15). If your hamstrings are relatively flexible, you may be able to get your right leg to 90 degrees. If not, don't be discouraged. Your goal is to increase your flexibility, slowly and smoothly.

Hold this stretch for 20 seconds. Remember to keep your back flat on the mat by contracting your gluteal and abdominal muscles. Return to the starting position. Repeat this exercise with the other leg. Hold for 20 seconds. Repeat this entire procedure 3 times. This exercise stretches the hamstrings, and it also stretches the calf muscles and strengthens the hip flexors, gluteal muscles, and abdominal muscles.

▶ **Quadriceps stretch:**

Stand in front of a chair or wall. With your left hand, support yourself on the wall or chair. Bend your right knee and grab your right ankle with your right hand behind you. Pull your right ankle backward so that you feel a stretch in the front of your right thigh.

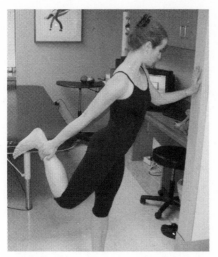

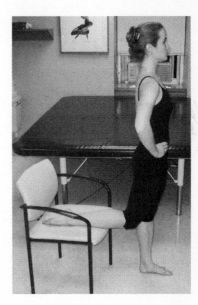

13.16

13.17

Don't pull your right ankle directly up to your right buttock. Instead, concentrate on pulling it up toward the ceiling and backward away from your buttocks (Figure 13.16). This way you won't compress your right knee too much and overstress the cartilage and other structures in your knee. If this pose is difficult, an alternate method is to place a chair behind you and bend your right knee so that your right shin rests on the chair (Figure 13.17). (You can place a pillow or cushion on the chair for comfort.) The point is to feel the stretch in the front of your left thigh. Hold for 20 seconds. Repeat on the other side. Hold for 20 seconds. Repeat the entire procedure 2 times.

▶ **Hip flexor stretch:**

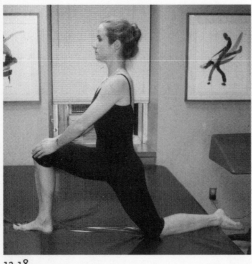

13.18

The hip flexors are also in the front of your thigh, but they are a bit higher up than the quadriceps. The quadriceps stretch will partially stretch these muscles. Another good way to stretch them—and that will also stretch the quadriceps—is to kneel on both knees. Now, bend your right leg in front of you with the knee flexed to 90 degrees. Don't let your right knee bend forward past the toes of your right foot as you flex the knee. Contract your abdominal muscles so that you keep your torso upright and straight (Figure 13.18). Feel the stretch in your left hip flexors. If you don't feel the stretch, you can slide your right foot out further in front of you so that you have to lean further into it. Your right knee should continue to be flexed at 90 degrees. The stretch should be in your left hip flexor. Hold the pose for 20 seconds. Repeat on the other side. Hold for 20 seconds. Repeat the entire procedure 3 times.

▸ **Calf and Achilles tendon stretch:**

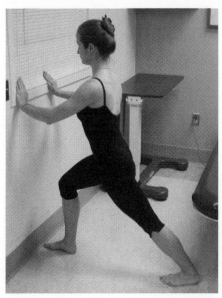

13.20

Stand facing the wall. Place both hands on the wall, with your left leg directly behind the right. Bend your right leg while keeping your left leg completely straight. Lean into the wall and push your left heel into the ground, feeling the stretch in the back of your left calf (Figure 13.20). As you do this, try to bring your toes up off the ground. If you do not feel the stretch, take a few steps back away from the wall and then lean in, repeating the above steps. Hold for 10–20 seconds. Repeat on the other side. Hold for 10–20 seconds. Repeat the entire procedure 3 times.

## Strengthening Exercises

Start by doing one of the following two versions of the squat. Pick the one that you find easiest.

▸ **The squat:**

This is a wonderful exercise for the quadriceps, hamstrings, and buttocks. If you can only do one exercise for your lower extremities, this would probably be the one. Stand with a chair behind you (or possibly without a chair once you are comfortable with the exercise), with your feet shoulder-width apart and firmly planted on the ground. At no time during this exercise should your feet leave the ground or should you elevate onto your toes. Your back should remain straight, and your abdominal muscles must remain contracted to help protect your lower back. Slowly bend your knees as if you were going to sit on the chair. Drop your buttocks straight backward and raise your arms up and forward to help with control and balance (Figure 15.1). Don't let your knees come forward past your toes. As you lower yourself, raise your arms up straight in front of you.

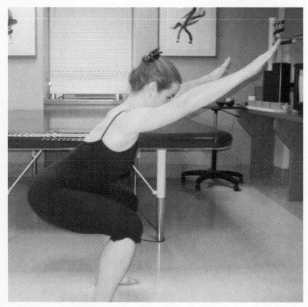

15.1

▶ **Modified squat:**

Alternatively, simply cross your arms across your chest so that your right hand holds your left shoulder and your left hand holds your right shoulder. As you lower yourself toward the chair, re-

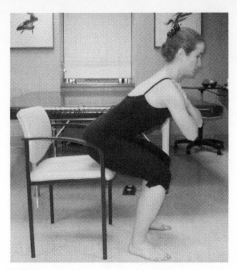

15.2

member to exhale (Figure 15.2). Before sitting in the chair, pause so that your thighs are parallel with the ground. Then, slowly stand up, keeping your abdominal muscles contracted and your back straight. This is one repetition of a true squat, but we call it a *modified squat* because, if you find it too difficult, you can place pillows on the chair. In this way, you lower yourself only to the pillows so that your thighs never become parallel with the floor. Start with as many pillows as you need. As you improve and become familiar with the mechanics of the exercise, you will need fewer and fewer pillows. Eventually, you should be able to get your thighs parallel (or close to parallel) with the floor. Again, the purpose of the exercise is not to "get parallel" but rather to strengthen your leg muscles.

Never sacrifice form to be able to lower yourself more. This exercise might feel awkward at first, but it will soon become easier. A doctor, physical therapist, or qualified trainer will be invaluable in helping you to perfect your form. Once you can do 4 sets of 12 repetitions without too much difficulty, you can progress to carrying 5–10 pound weights (or heavier) in your hands at your sides while doing the exercise. But first, perfect the exercise without any weight.

### ▶ Front of the thigh:

Sit in a chair with your feet dangling, but not touching the floor. You may need to use a pillow on the seat to lift yourself slightly higher. Make sure you are secure in your seat so you won't fall off. Grip the sides of the chair for support (Figure 15.3A). With your feet pointing only slightly outward to the sides, slowly extend your left leg (Figure 15.3B). Remember to exhale as you do this. Don't

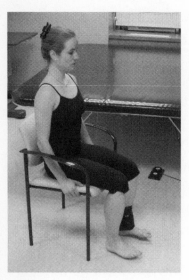
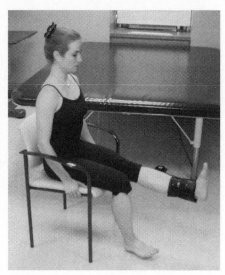

15.3A 15.3B

lock your knee. Extend it so that it is almost completely straight, but not quite. Pause and slowly flex your knee so it returns to the starting position. Next, do the same with your right knee. Perform three sets. If you find this exercise easy, attach a 2-pound ankle weight (which you can purchase at any exercise equipment store). Increase the weight when you can do 3 sets of 12 repetitions.

▶ **Outside of the hip:**

Lie on the exercise mat on your left side and bend your left knee so that your foot is behind you. Keep your right leg straight (Figure 15.7A). Slowly raise your right leg up in the air, so that it makes about a 45-degree angle with your body (Figure 15.7B). Feel the squeeze in the outside of your hip. Pause, and allow your leg to come down so that it aligns with your body. If possible, do not allow your right leg to lower all the way to the floor (Figure 15.7C). Instead, pause when it aligns with your body, and then raise it again to 45 degrees. Repeat this for 8–12 repetitions. If you can't stop your leg when it aligns with your body, allow it to slowly lower to the ground and then repeat. Turn onto your right side and repeat the

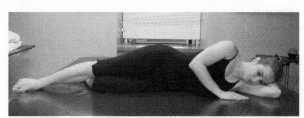

15.7A

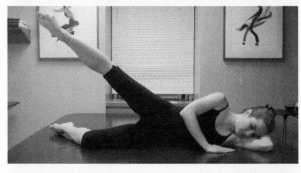

15.7B

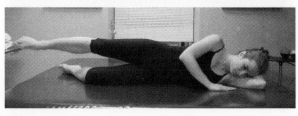

15.7C

exercise with your left leg. Once you can do 3 sets of 12 repetitions, add 2-pound ankle weights.

Now, repeat the stretching exercises that you did before. Follow this with 30-minutes of aerobic exercise, if possible. Good aerobic exercises include using an elliptical machine or swimming. Try to avoid jogging during the beginning of the rehabilitation process, because the constant pounding can be hard on your joints.

Stop and call your doctor if you experience any nausea, vomiting, headaches, chest pain, significant shortness of breath, or other medical problems while exercising.

## Arthritis of the Hip

Every exercise plan must address endurance, flexibility, and strength. Start each workout routine with a 5–10 minute warm-up, which may be as simple as going for a brisk walk. The point is to get your blood pumping and your heart rate up. Never exercise through joint pain; if your joint hurts, stop and rest, and then gradually ease back into the exercise. If the pain persists, talk to your doctor. You may need to take a mild pain reliever before exercising and ice the painful joint after exercising. Even if the joint is not painful immediately after exercising, ice is a powerful anti-inflammatory. A simple way to ice a joint is to put a bag of frozen peas on the joint for 15–20 minutes. If you have diabetes or any problem with your nerves that make it difficult to feel heat or cold, be careful to not keep the frozen peas (or ice) on for too long, to avoid injuring your skin.

This exercise program involves 4 stretches and 5 strengthening exercises.

## BEGIN WITH THESE STRETCHES:

▶ **Hamstring stretch:**

Stand with your legs shoulder-width apart and bend forward slowly, keeping your entire back and knees straight, and bending only from your hips. Reach out for the

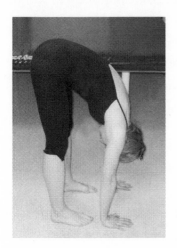

ground with your palms down, trying to touch the floor (Figure 13.13). Feel the stretch in the back of your thighs. Take it very slowly at first, and remember to feel the stretch but don't cause pain. (Don't sacrifice form for increased "motion.") If you bend from your lower back or bend your knees, you will certainly be able to reach lower. However, the purpose of this exercise is to stretch the hamstrings in

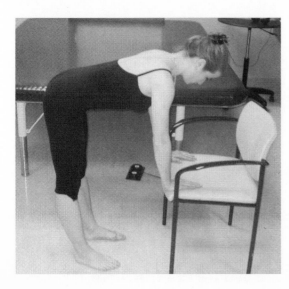

ABOVE: 13.13
LEFT: 13.14

the back of your thighs, not necessarily to actually reach the floor. Bending your knees and/or lower back will only stress these joints and will not help stretch your hamstrings.

Some people, who can't come this close to the floor, find it helpful to perform a modified version of this stretch. To do this, place a chair in front of you and reach down for the chair (Figure 13.14). If you can't reach the chair without breaking form, place pillows on the chair until you can reach over and touch the pillows, bending only from the hips. As you become more flexible, you will be able to remove the pillows from the chair. Eventually, you will be able to forgo the chair and reach down to your ankles, and perhaps your feet and even the floor.

▶ **Another hamstring stretch:**

Try this hamstring stretch if your lower back hurts. Lie on your back with your legs fully extended. Flatten your back so there is no space between your lumbar spine and the mat. You can do this by contracting your gluteal muscles (also called *glutes* or *buttocks*) to raise

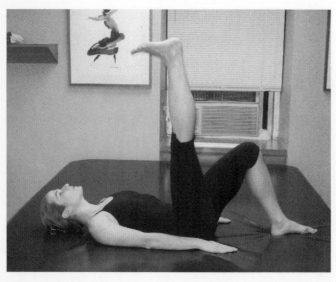

13.15

them slightly off the mat. You should also contract your abdominal muscles, pushing your belly button into the mat. This is a good strengthening exercise that will help protect your lower back.

Next, bend your left knee so that your left foot is flat on the mat. Now, lift your right leg up to the ceiling, keeping your leg completely straight and your ankle bent. Lift your leg as far as it will go (Figure 13.15). If your hamstrings are relatively flexible, you may be able to get your right leg to 90 degrees. If not, don't be discouraged. Your goal is to increase your flexibility, slowly and smoothly. Hold this stretch for 20 seconds. Remember to keep your back flat on the mat by contracting your gluteal and abdominal muscles. Return to the starting position. Repeat this exercise with the other leg. Hold for 20 seconds. Repeat this entire procedure 3 times. This exercise stretches the hamstrings, and it also stretches the calf muscles and strengthens the hip flexors, gluteal muscles, and abdominal muscles.

▶ **Quadriceps stretch:**

13.16

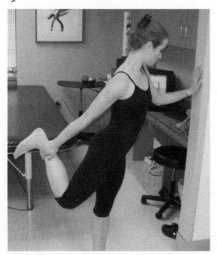

Stand in front of a chair or wall. With your left hand, support yourself using the wall or chair. Bend your right knee and grab your right ankle with your right hand behind you. Pull your right ankle backward so that you feel a stretch in the front of your right thigh. Don't pull your right ankle directly up to your right buttock. Instead, concentrate on pulling

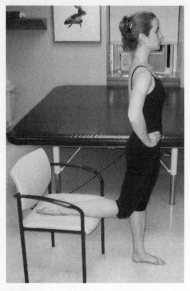

13.17

your left ankle up toward the ceiling and backward away from your buttocks (Figure 13.16). This way you won't compress your right knee too much and overstress the cartilage and other structures in your knee. If this pose is difficult, an alternate method is to place a chair behind you and bend your right knee so that your right shin rests on the chair (Figure 13.17). (You can place a pillow or cushion on the chair for comfort.) The point is to feel the stretch in the front of your left thigh. Hold for 20 seconds. Repeat on the other side. Hold for 20 seconds. Repeat the entire procedure 2 times.

▶ **Hip flexor stretch:**

The hip flexors are also in the front of your thigh, but they are a bit higher up than the quadriceps. The quadriceps stretch will partially stretch these muscles. Another good way to stretch them—and that will also stretch the quadriceps— is to kneel on both knees. Now, bend your right leg in front of you with the knee flexed to 90 degrees. Don't let your right knee bend forward past the toes of your right foot as you flex the knee. Contract your abdominal muscles so that you keep your torso upright and straight (Figure 13.18). Feel the stretch in your left hip flexors. If you don't feel the stretch, you can slide your right foot out further in front of you so that you have to lean further into it. Your right knee should continue to be flexed at 90 degrees. The stretch should be in your left hip flexor. Hold the pose for 20 seconds. Repeat on the other side. Hold for 20 seconds.

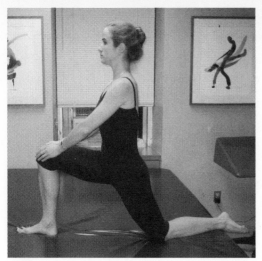

Repeat the entire procedure 3 times.

13.18

▶ **Piriformis stretch:**

The piriformis is one of the muscles in the hip area, and it is common for it to become tight. Lie on your back with both knees bent to 90 degrees. Place your right foot in front of your left knee so that it comes to rest on the knee. Next, gently pull your left thigh toward your chest, feeling the stretch in the back of your right buttock (Figure 13.19). This may be an awkward position to get into at first, but it is a wonderful stretch, once you understand how to

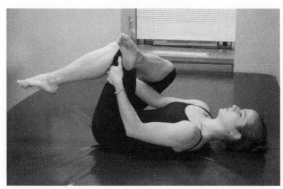

13.19

do it. Remember, stretching should not be painful, so stop if it is. However, try to go slowly, and gently move until you feel the stretch in the back of your buttock. Hold the pose for 20 seconds. Repeat on the other side. Hold for 20 seconds. Repeat the entire procedure 3 times.

## STRENGTHENING

Start by doing one of the following two versions of the squat. Pick the one that you find easiest.

▶ **The squat:**

This is a wonderful exercise for the quadriceps, hamstrings, and buttocks. If you can only do one exercise for your lower extremities, this would probably be the one. Stand with a chair behind you (or possibly without a chair once you are comfortable with the exercise), with your feet shoulder-width apart and firmly planted

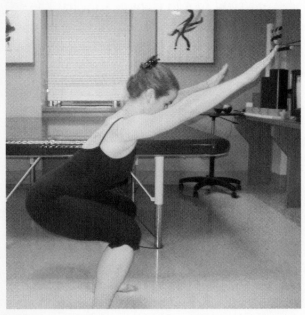

15.1

on the ground. At no time during this exercise should your feet leave the ground or should you elevate onto your toes. Your back should remain straight, and your abdominal muscles must remain contracted to help protect your lower back. Slowly bend your knees as if you were going to sit on the chair. Drop your buttocks straight backward and raise your arms up and forward to help with control and balance (Figure 15.1). Don't let your knees come forward past your toes. As you lower yourself, raise your arms up straight in front of you.

▶ **Modified Squat:**

Alternatively, simply cross your arms across your chest so that your right hand holds your left shoulder and your left hand holds your right shoulder. As you lower yourself toward the chair, remember to exhale (Figure 15.2). Before sitting in the chair, pause so that your thighs are parallel with the ground. Then, slowly stand up, keeping your abdominal muscles contracted and your back straight. This is one repetition of a true squat, but we call it a *modified squat* because

15.2

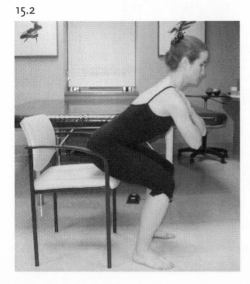

if you find it too difficult, you can place pillows on the chair. In this way, you lower yourself only to the pillows so that your thighs never become parallel with the floor. Start with as many pillows as you need. As you improve and become familiar with the mechanics of the exercise, you will need fewer and fewer pillows. Eventually, you should be able to get your thighs parallel (or close to parallel) with the floor. Again, the purpose of the exercise is not to "get parallel" but rather to strengthen your leg muscles.

Never sacrifice form to be able to lower yourself more. This exercise might feel awkward at first, but it will soon become easier. A doctor, physical therapist, or qualified trainer will be invaluable in helping you to perfect your form. Once you can do 4 sets of 12 repetitions without too much difficulty, you can progress to carrying 5–10 pound weights (or heavier) in your hands at your sides while doing the exercise. But first, perfect the exercise without any weight.

▶ **Back of the hip:**

Lie on an exercise mat with your stomach on the mat. You may use one pillow to rest your head on and another to support your pelvis (Figure 15.6A). Keeping your legs straight, raise your right leg off the mat (Figure 15.6B). Feel the squeeze in your buttocks. Pause,

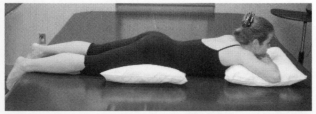

15.6A

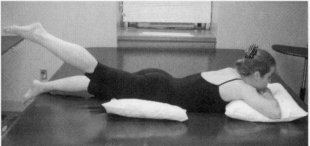

15.6B

then slowly lower your leg to the mat. Repeat with your left leg. As you improve, you may need to use ankle weights to increase resistance. Placing a pillow beneath your pelvis can make this exercise more comfortable. Perform 3 sets of 12 repetitions on both sides.

▶ **Outside of the hip:**

Lie on the exercise mat on your left side. Bend your left knee so that your foot is behind you. Keep your right leg straight (Figure 15.7A). Slowly raise your right leg up in the air, so that it makes about a 45-degree angle with your body (Figure15.7B). Feel the squeeze in the outside of your hip. Pause, and allow your leg to align with your body. If possible, do not allow your right leg to lower all the

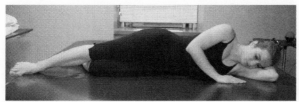

15.7A

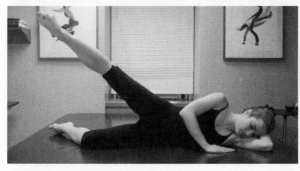

15.7B

way to the floor (Figure 15.17C). Instead, pause when it aligns with your body, and then raise it again to 45 degrees. Repeat this for 8–12 repetitions. If you can't stop your leg when it aligns with your body, allow it to slowly lower to the ground and then repeat. Turn onto

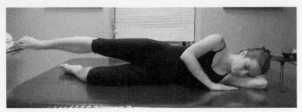

15.7C

your right side and repeat the exercise with your left leg. Once you can do 3 sets of 12 repetitions, add 2-pound ankle weights.

▶ **Inner thigh:**

A good way to exercise the inside of your thighs is to lie on your back with your feet straight up in the air so that your hips are bent at approximately 90 degrees. It's okay if you need to bend your knees slightly (Figure 15.8A). Allow your legs to slowly fall to the sides so that they make a V in the air. Pause when you feel a slight stretch in your inner thighs—this should occur when your thighs form approximately a 60–90 degree angle, depending on your flexibility (Figure 15.8B). After a brief pause, squeeze your thighs together to bring your legs back to midline. Pause and repeat. Do 3 sets

15.8A

15.8B

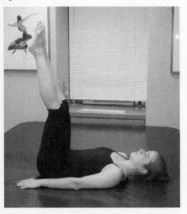
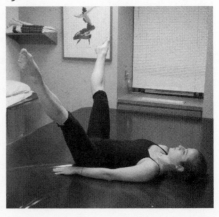

of 12 repetitions. If your back hurts while doing this exercise, try doing a posterior pelvic tilt at the same time (see core strengthening for details on how to do this). If your pain persists, try using your hands to support your buttocks. If pain persists despite these modifications, stop the exercise.

## CORE STRENGTHENING

▶ **Posterior pelvic tilt:**

This is perhaps the best and safest way for many people to exercise their abdominal muscles. Start by lying on your back on an exercise mat or carpet. Bend your knees so your feet are flat on the mat (Figure 15.10A). Squeeze your gluteal muscles together so they rise slightly off the mat. At the same time, contract your abdominal muscles. The curve in your lumbar spine should straighten, and your lower back should be flat against the mat (Figure 15.10B). If you are not sure, check your position by trying to place your hand underneath your lower back. In this position, you should not be able to do this. Next, bring both knees to your chest. Then straighten your right leg while keeping your left knee at your chest with about 90-degree flexion in the hip (Figure 15.10C). Next,

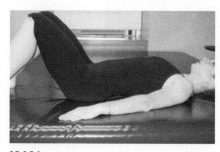

15.10A

15.10B

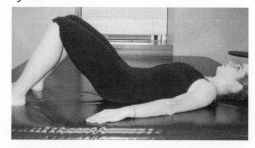

bend your right leg so that your right knee comes to your chest, and then straighten your left leg. It is as if you are lying on the ground and riding a bicycle in midair with your gluteal and abdominal muscles contracted to reverse the lumbar curve and protect your back. This is a challenging activity. At first, you might only be able

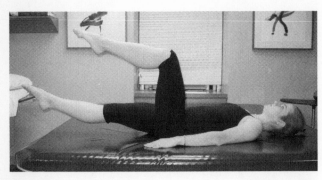

15.10C

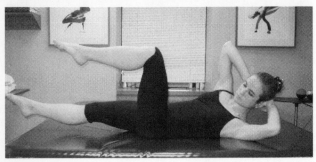

15.10D

to straighten your lumbar curve. After you can straighten your lumbar curve easily, begin to bend and straighten your legs. When you can do 3 sets of 12 repetitions while bending and straightening your legs, you can begin to bring your arms into the exercise. Do this by folding your arms behind your head. As you bring your right knee to your chest, move your left elbow toward the right knee. Then repeat with your left knee and right elbow (Figure 15.10D). Most importantly, continue to squeeze your gluteal and abdominal muscles so that your back remains flat on the mat, reversing the lumbar curve. As always, do not sacrifice your form. The form in this exercise requires particularly attention to detail, and physician or trainer instruction and guidance is strongly recommended.

▸ **Core strengthening with the "bridge":**

With your knees bent at a 45-degree angle and your feet flat on the ground, contract your gluteal and abdominal muscles and raise your abdomen and buttocks off the ground so that your body is straight from your chest to your knees (Figure 15.12). This is an excellent exercise for your core muscles as well as your glutes. Concentrate on keeping your abdominals and gluteal muscles contracted and tight at all times during the exercise. It may help to think of driving your heels into the ground. (Some people call this a *bridge*.) Hold this position for 10 seconds. Repeat 3 times.

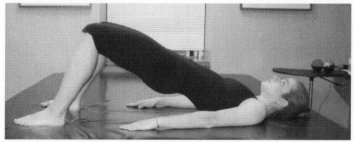

15.12

Follow these core strengthening exercises with 30 minutes of aerobics, if possible. Good aerobic exercises include using an elliptical machine or swimming. Try to avoid jogging during the beginning of your rehabilitation process because the constant pounding on the ground can be hard on your joints. Finally, repeat the stretching exercises that you did at the beginning of your workout.

Stop and call your doctor if you experience any nausea, vomiting, headache, chest pain, significant shortness of breath, or other medical problems while exercising.

# 18

# Achieving Lasting Lifestyle Changes

I HAVE ALWAYS appreciated the advice my cousin John gave me when I was in grade school: "At the end of the day, there is only you. That's it. You have to look in the mirror and live with yourself."

This is simple advice, but powerful, and I've never forgotten it. It applies to every facet of life, including what you do behind closed doors, the thoughts you allow to ruminate in your mind, how you treat your neighbors, the way you interact with others, the way you interact with nature, and the way you approach something that no one else can truly understand as well as you can: your pain. Only you know when you're in pain. Only you can take the necessary steps to relieve yourself of the pain and stiffness of arthritis, and prevent it from coming back. Of course, you need help. That's why you're reading this book. It's also why you need the love and support of family and friends. However, the ultimate responsibility for your success or failure lies with you.

Often our best intentions go unfulfilled. Some of the common complaints I hear from patients include:

"I really want to exercise. I know I have to. I just never have time."

"I have so many responsibilities. By the end of the day, I just don't have the energy to exercise."

"I try to follow my diet, but at the end of the day I want comfort food."

"I start by eating one cookie, just for a little treat, but then I end up eating the whole bag."

Intentions are important, but results are what count. Results come from two inner resources: purpose and discipline.

Purpose is more than just intent. You may *want* to have a better diet, exercise more, and take your daily supplements. However, without a sense of purpose and deeper meaning behind your intentions, you have little chance of achieving the discipline required to fulfill your goals. Purpose carries with it a sense of fulfillment. To find your purpose, you must first identify your core set of values—the principles by which you live your life. This is imperative if you truly want to accomplish lasting change.

If you are reading this book, it is likely that one of your core values is to stay healthy. For some people, staying healthy is important because they want to live long enough to spend more high-functioning quality time with their family and loved ones. For others, staying healthy is simply an inherent value, important in and of itself.

Once you have identified good health as a core value, you will have identified the reservoir of meaning from which you will derive purpose for specific actions. With the knowledge that you have gained from this book, and from talking with your physician, you know the steps you need to take in order to achieve and maintain better health, particularly when it comes to arthritis. Therefore, your purpose for these specific actions is obvious.

Next comes discipline, undeniably the workhorse that lets you accomplish your goals, but not in the way you might suspect. There is a permeating sense in our society that you can make yourself do anything if you have enough discipline. This is a myth, at least in part. In fact, the discipline needed to change our behavior patterns is enormous. Just as a balloon can hold only so much air—or a bottle only so much water—our bodies have a limited amount of energy available on a daily basis. In fact, energy is a precious personal commodity.

It takes a tremendous amount of willpower to undertake a new behavior, even a relatively small one. Therefore, it is important that you learn to invest your energy carefully. Use self-discipline to follow the course of action that will best help you create healthy habits, one at a time. Once a new activity has become a habit, it requires very little energy and discipline to maintain it. You don't need discipline to *continue* a habit. You need it to *break* a habit. Use your energy and discipline to routinely break bad habits, and replace them with new, healthier ones. In this way, you will eventually make major, sustainable changes.

Consider the goal of eating a healthy breakfast of fruits and vegetables, instead of the large cup of coffee and pastry (filled with omega-6 saturated fats) that you usually get on the way to the office. The first step is to develop your purpose and a plan. Your purpose is to eat healthy because it is consistent with your core value of staying healthy. Your plan is to have a bowl of fruit and a glass of water before leaving for work. The next step is to avoid coffee and pastry. To fulfill the first part of your plan, you purchase plenty of delicious fruits and vegetables. You even invest in a water filter that you can easily attach to your sink so you have filtered water.

The next step is to put your plan into daily action. You wake up and will yourself to eat a bowl of fruit and drink a tall glass of filtered water. More than likely, you are surprised by how much you enjoy your new breakfast. However, when you get to work, you still crave pastry and coffee, because fats and caffeine have addictive qualities. Breaking these kinds of habits is the key to successfully improving your health. If you find it extremely difficult to do without coffee, try switching to tea, which has less caffeine and contains beneficial antioxidants.

You have used precious mental energy and successfully willed yourself to eat a healthy breakfast, rather than an unhealthy one. When it's time for lunch, you might be able to will yourself to again choose a healthy meal. However, each time you pass the vending machine, it becomes harder to ignore the tasty treats. Your habit of using sugary, fat-filled, comfort foods to alleviate stress is hard to ignore. Even if you can ignore it, dinner is coming, and it will be extremely hard to will yourself to eat a healthy dinner, because your energy resources are becoming depleted. If you do manage to eat a healthy dinner, you will be that much more hard-pressed to avoid an unhealthy, late-night snack. In addition, if you have forced yourself to eat healthy all day—when normally you don't—it will be less likely that you will be able to discipline yourself to exercise.

## MAKE CHANGES GRADUALLY

Some people are able to eat healthy and exercise for several days, perhaps even for a few weeks. The trouble is that, for most of us, sudden major changes in behavior are not sustainable. How can behavior be changed in a sustainable way? The answer is by gradually changing, one habit at a time. As you make each new, healthy lifestyle change, you will realize that they add up quickly, and that each successive change becomes easier to make as you detoxify your body of old bad habits and replace them with healthy ones.

## TURNING GOOD HEALTH BEHAVIORS INTO HABITS

Habits are what you do without thinking about them. Many people consider themselves to be self-disciplined, and, in fact, they are. However, their ability to force themselves to act a certain way on a daily, sustained basis is based on their ability to learn new habits that, ironically, do not require self-discipline to maintain. These habits simply become a part of the day. Your day is full of rituals and habits. Brushing your teeth, for example, is a habit. You brush your teeth in the morning and before you go to bed. You don't have to force yourself or use self-discipline to brush your teeth; you brush them because *not* doing it feels wrong. Similarly, as you practice new lifestyle behaviors, such as eating healthy and exercising, *not* doing these things will also feel wrong. Then, you will have achieved lasting change.

# PART IV.

## Supplements

People have been using plants for medicinal purposes since the dawn of civilization. In the code of Hammurabi in Babylon, circa 1770 BC, and in ancient Egypt, circa 1550 BC, records show that people used plants for healing. Pharmaceutical companies didn't invent drugs—they just brilliantly and meticulously systematized the process.

Take aspirin, for example. As far back as 460-377 BC, Hippocrates noted that the leaves of white willow bark (*Salix alba*) helped alleviate pain, and he prescribed chewing these leaves to women in labor. In North America, white willow bark was used for centuries by Native Americans to treat fever and pain, but it wasn't until the 1820s that European scientists began actively studying the chemical properties of plants and discovered that salicin was the active component in willow. They soon realized that salicin was irritating to the stomach. In 1853, Charles Frederic Gerhardt, a French scientist, combined sodium salicylate with acetyl chloride. The sodium neutralized the salicylic acid and made it less irritating to the stomach.

For reasons that are unclear, Gerhardt abandoned his research. More than 30 years later, Felix Hoffman, an employee of Friedrich Bayer and Company, found a way to produce a pure, stable form of salicin—acetylsalicylic acid—that was less irritating to the stomach. Felix tested his discovery on his father, who was suffering from arthritis. In 1899, the Bayer company trademarked "Aspirin," the first major medicine to be made available in tablet form.

## THE COMPLEXITIES OF DRUG DEVELOPMENT

The process of identifying and then turning a naturally occurring compound in a plant or herb into a drug for consumption and sale is time- and labor-intensive, and also extremely costly. Of every 10,000 compounds analyzed, perhaps only one will make it to market, and the process may take 10–15 years, or more. According to a report by the Tufts Center for the Study of Drug Development, the cost of bringing a new drug to market in the late 1990s was $897 million, which is double the average of bringing a new drug to market in the 1980s, and five times the cost in the 1970s. Drug companies now report that bringing a single new drug to market costs in excess of $1 billion dollars.

An abundance of naturally occurring substances with significant potential healing powers have not yet been made available in pill form. They can be found in our own backyards, the Amazon rain forest, African jungles, and the flora of the deep sea. The immense cost in work hours and dollars to bring any of these unknown compounds out of their natural habitat and into a laboratory to be extracted, analyzed, tested on animals, eventually tested on humans, and finally made ready for sale, is almost overwhelming. Some compounds have been identified and analyzed, but they have not yet been put through the rigors of clinical testing required for Food and Drug Administration (FDA) approval. Some of these substances are marketed as nutritional or herbal supplements.

In 1994, the United States Congress passed a law defining nutritional supplements, and requiring them to be labeled as dietary supplements and identified as not intended to be a substitute for certain foods. A nutritional supplement can be defined as a product intended for consumption in tablet, capsule, powder, soft gel, gel cap, or liquid form, and containing vitamin(s), mineral(s), herb(s), other botanicals, amino acids, or any combination thereof. Because they are regulated by the FDA as foods, and not drugs, nutritional supplements are not subject to the same rigorous testing standards as drugs (including over-the-counter drugs) in terms of manufacturing process, safety, and efficacy. The active ingredient(s) in a nutritional supplement may not be fully understood or even known. Some supplements have been shown to have different ingredients from those they advertise. Some have even been found to contain harmful substances in the forms of microorganisms, prescription drug ingredients, and metals.

When the federal government identifies companies making inappropriate, dangerous, deceptive, or unsubstantiated claims, it can take action against them. However, government oversight, even of misleading and disreputable sellers, remains limited because of the enormous amount of money needed (several billion dollars annually) and the large number of small companies involved. The lack of precision of descriptive terms, which allows disreputable businesses to mislead and misguide the public without doing anything "illegal," makes it even more difficult for the government to maintain control. Because the terms commonly used for advertising supplements have no legal definition, a company can advertise that its formula uses a "standardized" process that has been "verified," or even "certified," without these terms meaning anything of substance.

Although supplements do not need to meet the same rigorous standards as drugs, there are ways to verify that a supplement has met some standards. For example, the "USP Dietary Supplement Verified" seal indicates that a supplement has met certain basic manufacturing standards. Groups such as ConsumerLab.com and NSF International evaluate drugs and make their evaluations available. If you choose to take supplements, it is best to get them from a reputable company that has been in business for some time and has good ratings from such independent organizations.

Given the large number of supplements on the market, the claims being made, and the volume of advertising, it can be confusing for a person with arthritis who is trying to decide which supplements, if any, are right for them. Research substantiates possibly taking 3–4 supplements if you have arthritis. In addition to a multivitamin each day (which everyone should take) you should probably be taking glucosamine, chondroitin, fish oils, and cherry supplements. Two other supplements worth considering are avocado soybean unsaponifiables (ASU) and methylsulfonylmethane (MSM). These supplements are explained in detail in Chapter 20.

## Cautions about Supplements

Supplements can be very helpful for some people, but there are some basic precautions:

- Always talk with your doctor before taking any supplement.

- If you are pregnant, planning to become pregnant, nursing, or under the age of 18, do not take the supplements recommended in this book.

- Ask your doctor to monitor you with regular blood, kidney, and liver function tests while you are taking supplements.

If you are taking aspirin, blood thinners, or any herbs, tell your doctor. Some supplements may thin the blood, and some can interfere with the action of the prescribed medications you are already taking.

# Chapter 19.

## Glucosamine and Chondroitin Sulfate

Gᴌᴜᴄᴏsᴀᴍɪɴᴇ ɪs an "amino sugar" that consists of glucose (sugar) and glutamine, an amino acid. From a biomechanical standpoint, glucosamine helps cartilage hold water, which is vital to its health. Glucosamine stimulates chondrocytes, the cells in the joint that produce cartilage. The more glucosamine that is available in the joint, the more cartilage the joint will be able to produce, the more the cartilage will be able to hold onto water, and the less likely it will be broken down and metabolized.

Glucosamine also has anti-inflammatory properties, including inhibition of the COX-2 enzyme. The COX-2 inhibitors, including Celebrex®, Vioxx®, and Bextra®, are targeted to relieve the pain and inflammation of conditions such as arthritis. However, Vioxx® and Bextra® have such potentially severe side effects that they have been taken off the market. Celebrex® also has potentially significant side effects.

Chondroitin is a long chain of sugars that helps cartilage hold water. It is derived from animal tissues, particularly ligaments, tendons, bone ends, and joint capsules. Chondroitin also inhibits cartilage metabolism. Like glucosamine, chondroitin has anti-inflammatory properties. It stimulates the production of cartilage and hyaluronic acid, an important component of joint fluid.

## REDUCING THE SYMPTOMS OF ARTHRITIS

From a conceptual and biochemical standpoint, both glucosamine and chondroitin should be helpful for the symptoms and disease process of arthritis. What is truly impressive is the increasing clinical evidence showing their efficacy in reducing both symptoms and the need for medication. Numerous studies, including long-term, placebo-controlled studies—the "gold standard" in clinical study design—and "meta-analyses" that review all of the published data, have demonstrated the effectiveness of glucosamine and chondroitin, earning them a place in the treatment regimen of patients with arthritis.

In four key studies, glucosamine taken alone was shown to be as effective, or more so, than anti-inflammatory medications such as ibuprofen. In each study, glucosamine was found to be safer and without the negative side effects of anti-inflammatory medication.

A study sponsored by the National Institutes of Health (NIH) confirmed the benefit of taking glucosamine and chondroitin together. "The Glucosamine/Chondroitin Arthritis Intervention Trial (GAIT)" was anticipated to be the definitive study on glucosamine and chondroitin. In fact, for the most part it simply confirmed what many people already knew. The study compared taking glucosamine alone, chondroitin alone, and glucosamine and chondroitin together, to placebo and celecoxib (Celebrex®) for painful arthritis of the knee. The results showed that glucosamine and chondroitin were effective when taken alone for the treatment of moderate-to-severe arthritis of the knee. When taken together, they were even more effective, including more effective than celecoxib. The relatively high placebo rate may have made it difficult for the study to detect a statistically significant difference in people with mild symptoms.

Glucosamine and chondroitin also modify the underlying disease process of arthritis because they delay narrowing of the joint space and the degradation of cartilage, as well as stimulating new cartilage growth. For an aging population that is looking for ways to slow or reverse joint damage, this is promising news, indeed.

It's unclear how glucosamine and chondroitin actually reach the joint, and future research might modify the current recommendations. However, with the positive research results already available—especially in the absence of apparent serious side effects as compared with over-the-counter anti-inflammatory drugs and prescription medications—it is reasonable to include glucosamine and chondroitin as front-line supplements in the treatment of arthritis.

The abundance of research has primarily focused on the use of these supplements in the treatment of arthritis of the knee. The results obtained from taking glucosamine and chondroitin for arthritis of the knee are not necessarily applicable to other parts of the body, such as the hip, although it is not known why. Further studies are needed to address this issue.

## Choosing a Source of Glucosamine and Chondroitin Sulfate

Glucosamine supplements are available in one of three forms: glucosamine hydrochloride, N-acetyl glucosamine, and glucosamine sulfate. Most clinical studies used glucosamine sulfate, and this is the recommended form. Glucosamine sulfate can and should be taken in combination with chondroitin sulfate. The pill form is preferred, rather than the liquid. Most of the studies used pills, which are generally less expensive and possibly easier for the body to absorb.

The recommended dosage for glucosamine is 1,500 mg daily; chondroitin is 800–1,200 mg daily. They can be taken once daily or divided into 2–3 equal doses. When taken once a day, more of the supplements actually reach your bloodstream and, presumably, your joints.

It is important to purchase supplements only from reputable companies. Some reports have revealed that as little as 1 out of 15 products on the market may actually contain the amount of glucosamine they claim. It is also important to look for the exact content of glucosamine and chondroitin. Some companies advertise "glucosamine complex" or "chondroitin complex," which may be diluted with other less expensive substances, or they may simply mix different types of glucosamine at smaller dosages. *Always look for the actual active ingredients in any supplement.*

Although there has been some concern that glucosamine might be contraindicated in people with diabetes, because it is partly a sugar, this appears not to be the case. Glucosamine does not appear to significantly raise blood glucose levels. Nevertheless, always discuss the risks and benefits of any new supplement with your physician and, in the case of glucosamine, monitor your blood sugar with your physician if you have diabetes.

Glucosamine is derived from the shells of shellfish such as lobster, crabs, and shrimp, and there is some concern that people with shellfish allergies should not take glucosamine. Although people with shellfish allergies are generally allergic to a protein in the meat of shellfish and not the shells themselves, it is possible that a piece of the meat could get into the shells during processing. If you have an allergy to shellfish, do not take glucosamine unless you have had a complete discussion of the risks with your personal physician. There are shellfish-free glucosamine products, and you and your physician can decide whether this is a good option.

# 20

# Fish Oil and Other Supplements

CHAPTER 8 considered the importance of consuming more foods containing omega-3 fatty acids. In other types of arthritis, such as rheumatoid arthritis and Raynaud's phenomenon, fish oil supplements have been shown to reduce symptoms to an extent similar to NSAIDs, but without their side effects. These results may or may not be generalized to osteoarthritis, but it would seem reasonable that they would help the inflammation of osteoarthritis, as well as that of other inflammatory joint conditions. Research also tends to indicate that fish oil supplements help with a variety of other ailments, including decreasing the risk of heart disease, cancer, diabetes, and depression.

Fish oil supplements or other omega-3 fatty acid supplements are not necessary if you already consume small, cold-water fish 2 or more times per week, and do not eat substantial amounts of saturated fats. If you do not eat enough fish, and are not a candidate for fish oil supplementation for any reason, evening primrose seed oil, borage seed oil, or flaxseed oil may be good substitutes. The important ingredient in these oils is gamma-linolenic acid (GLA). The typical suggested dose of GLA is 1,800 mg per day. Avoid taking GLA and fish oil supplements together. People who consume 3–4 servings of fish per week, but who also consume a substantial amount of omega-6 fatty acids in the form of red meat, can benefit from GLA supplementation. Of course, the best approach is to reduce your red meat consumption. However, if this not an option for you, consider these alternative supplements. Olive oil may also be beneficial. Be sure to discuss the options with your physician before taking supplements, because they might be contraindicated for medical conditions you have, or interact with prescription medications you are already taking.

If you do not consume at least 3–4 servings of small, cold-water fish per week, and if you have no contraindications, I recommend taking mercury-free fish oil supplements. Of course, it would be better if you started eating more small, cold-water fish. The omega-3 fatty acids eicosapentaenoic acid (EPA) and docosahexaenoic acid (DHA) are the important ingredients in fish oil supplements. Most physicians recommend taking 3,000 mg of EPA/DHA per day. As with all supplements, be sure to read the label on the bottle to ensure that you are actually getting enough EPA/DHA. Some companies advertise "1,000 mg of fish oil," but when you read more closely, you will learn that there are actually only 300 mg of EPA/DHA and the rest is filler. Also, be sure to buy only reputable brands. A month of high quality fish oil supplements can cost as much as $45.

## Mercury Contamination of Fish Oil Supplements

Most studies show that mercury contamination is not an issue with reputable brands of fish oil supplements. If you are concerned about the possibility of contamination, look for brands that state on the label that they are mercury-free. Also, to limit the risk of taking excessive amounts of vitamin A and possibly other vitamins, look for fish oil supplements derived from the fleshy body of the fish, not from the liver.

Omega-3 fatty acids are susceptible to degradation caused by heat, light, and oxygen. Whether in tablet or liquid form, supplements should be sold in dark bottles and stored in dark containers, tightly sealed, in a refrigerator, freezer, or other cool, dark, dry place.

EPA/DHA and GLA oils thin the blood. If you bleed easily, have a diagnosed bleeding disorder, are taking a blood-thinning medication, discuss their risks and benefits with your physician. Because of their ability to thin the blood, combining different omega-3 fatty acid supplements is not recommended, though occasionally it might be warranted. Note that NSAIDs, such as ibuprofen and naproxen, also increase clotting time.

The more common side effects of fish oil supplements include a "fishy" smelling burp or taste in the mouth, or slight gastrointestinal upset and gas. If you experience any of these mild symptoms, discuss them with your doctor and consider decreasing the dosage to 1,000 mg of EPA/DHA. You can slowly increase the dosage back to 3,000 mg per day as your symptoms resolve.

## Cherries, Avocado Soybean Unsaponifiables (ASU), and Methylsulfonylmethane (MSM)

This section focuses on three additional supplements: cherries, avocado soybean unsaponifiables (ASU), and methylsulfonylmethane (MSM). These supplements have some positive attributes and might ease the symptoms of arthritis, but their effectiveness is not as well supported as that of glucosamine, chondroitin, and fish oil.

### Cherries

Cherries are a traditional folk medicine remedy for arthritis. They are rich in antioxidants such as flavonoids (including quercetin, a flavonoid that is believed to have particularly potent antioxidant activity), vitamin C, and beta-carotene. Several studies have shown that consuming 20 cherries per day might be as effective in relieving pain as medications such as aspirin, and several studies have suggested a decrease in blood levels of uric acid, which can precipitate an attack of gout, an arthritis-like disorder. Blood markers for inflammation also tended to drop.

Although cherries can be obtained from your diet, the quantities needed to show an effect are higher than may be reasonable to consume—up to half a pound or more per day or as one or more glasses of cherry juice. Additionally, they may not be available much of the year, and may have more calories than are good for you.

If you area unable to get cherries or cherry juice from your diet, a supplement is recommended. Cherry supplements are available in both liquid and capsule forms. The recommended dosage is 2,000 mg per day of cherry fruit extract, taken in 2–4 divided dosages.

### Avocado Soybean Unsaponifiables (ASU)

*Avocado soybean unsaponifiables* (ASU) has been prescribed in France as *A1S2* or *piascledine* since the early 1990s for managing the symptoms of arthritis. *Saponification* is the chemical process of making soap from oil and lye, and these unsaponifiables are the approximately 1% portion of the oil from avocados and soybeans that cannot be made into soap. It is called *A1S2* because it comes from a mixture of 1 part avocado oil and 2 parts soybean oil.

A growing body of evidence shows that ASU stimulates the production of cartilage, inhibits its breakdown, and decreases pain to an extent similar to NSAIDs, but without negative side effects. Although side effects can include rash and migraine headaches, ASU is generally well tolerated. The most common side effect is a mildly upset stomach. The most common dosage of ASU is 300 mg, once per day. No additional benefit has been seen with higher dosages. One study found that patients with arthritis of the knee, who took 300 mg of ASU daily for 6 months, did not take less NSAIDs, but they did report significantly less pain and improved function after 2 months compared to patients who were given a placebo.

As with any supplement, ASU has the potential to interact with other medications. In particular, potential adverse reactions can occur with monoamine oxydase inhibitors (MAOIs), warfarin (Coumadin®), levothyroxine (thyroid hormone), and iron. Be sure to check with your physician before taking ASU.

### Methylsulfonylmethane (MSM)

Another supplement worth mentioning is methylsulfonylmethane (MSM), which is derived from dimethyl sulfoxide (DMSO). DMSO has been reported to be helpful for a variety of medical ailments, but it fell out of favor many years ago because of potential adverse reactions, including eye lens problems, and the fact that people who used it smelled like a mixture of garlic and oysters. MSM does not have these effects. Although the usefulness of MSM has not yet been proven, it has become popular.

If you are interested in trying MSM, discuss it first with your doctor; 500 mg twice per day is a reasonable amount. If you do not experience improvement after 12 weeks, discontinue its use. Further research may better define its role, if any, in the treatment of arthritis. The potential risks include headache, skin rash, and stomach upset. If you develop any of these symptoms, discontinue usage. Because MSM is relatively unstudied, there may be other unknown risks.

# PART V.

## Medical and Surgical Options

YOUR DOCTOR has many ways to help manage and relieve your arthritis symptoms. As discussed earlier, the most important initial task is to arrive at an accurate diagnosis. Joint pain can result from a variety of conditions, although the classic symptoms of pain and stiffness in the joints are most typically caused by arthritis. It is tempting to self-diagnose and then self-treat, but this is not advised. Self-diagnosis can be dangerous, because many other ailments can masquerade as arthritis.

A 66-year-old, overweight woman with pain and stiffness in her right knee that is worse in the morning and after prolonged activity probably has arthritis, but she might, for example, have a cancer with a metastasis to the knee or an infection in her knee joint. Either of these possibilities is unlikely, but a doctor should make that determination.

Almost every physician has at least one story that goes something like this: "I honestly thought he had arthritis, but I ordered an X-ray just to be safe. When I looked at the film, I saw a large lesion sitting right on the vertebral body. It turned out to be metastatic prostate cancer."

Your physician will take a full medical history, perform a physical examination, order any needed tests, arrive at an accurate diagnosis, and help you create a treatment plan that is right for you.

In addition to X-rays, CT scans, and/or MRIs, your doctor might order blood tests to help rule out infection, types of arthritis other than osteoarthritis, cancer, and other problems. Most people with straightforward signs and symptoms of arthritis may not require more than an X-ray. However, your physician will make that determination in order to help ensure that a more serious underlying disorder does not go undiagnosed and untreated.

Once a diagnosis has been made, your doctor has many treatments at his disposal. Exercise, diet, and supplementation offer the most lasting benefit. However, more invasive therapies such as medications, injections, and surgery are also available, and are sometimes necessary. Medications and injections often provide significant pain relief and allow you to participate in appropriate exercises so that the pain does not recur. Although it is the most invasive option, surgery has excellent results when used judiciously in the right circumstances and patients. It is helpful to understand your options, so you can have an educated discussion with your doctor about the different treatments available and make an informed decision about what would be best for you.

# 21.

## Medications

THREE TYPES of medications are available to treat arthritis:

▶ Topical (applied to the skin) pain-relieving medications
▶ Over-the-counter medications
▶ Prescription medications

None of these treatments can stop or reverse the process of arthritis, and anything you put on or into your body has potential side effects. Given this, you need to know why you should take a particular medication, what you can expect from it, and how and when you should use it.

Medications should be used in conjunction with diet, exercise, and supplementation. To illustrate this point, consider what would happen if all you did to manage your arthritis was take medication. If you have arthritis of the knee, for example, and you take extra-strength acetaminophen (Tylenol®) and do nothing else, what would happen? Your pain might improve because acetaminophen is a good *analgesic*, meaning it alleviates pain. However, the underlying disease process would not be affected. Your knee would continue to become more and more arthritic, because all you would be doing was blunting the pain. Gradually, the acetaminophen would stop controlling the pain and stiffness. At that point, you might begin to take a stronger pain medication, but your knee would continue to deteriorate.

## Brand Name or Generic?

The FDA regulates pharmaceutical manufacturers closely and, if a company claims its product has a certain amount of an active ingredient, then, according to the FDA, it does. Thus, buying the generic form of a medication should be just as good as buying a trade-name product. For example, acetaminophen is the active ingredient in Tylenol®. Most pharmacies sell their own brand of acetaminophen for a reduced price. Essentially, you are getting the same active ingredient at a discount. In theory, you should buy the generic form whenever possible.

In practice, however, some people report that they don't get as much relief unless they use the brand-name product. What should you do? Try it for yourself. If you need a pain reliever such as acetaminophen and cost is a concern, try the less expensive generic product first. The same is true for the NSAIDs, such as ibuprofen. The active ingredient ibuprofen is marketed under trade names such as Advil®, Motrin®, and Nuprin®. When shopping for an over-the-counter medication, look for the active ingredient, and then search next to it on the shelf for a generic drug with the same active ingredient at a lower price, and consider trying that one first.

## How Should I Use Medication?

Ideally, one reason that medications are prescribed is to allow you to participate pain-free in an active, structured physical therapy program, because strengthening and stretching the muscles that surround the joints will take the pressure off them. Additionally, you should alter your diet and take any appropriate supplements. By doing these things, you should be able to slowly taper off your pain medication instead of needing more and more of it. Medications and other pain-relieving procedures, such as injections, should be used as a bridge that allows you to proceed with your physical therapy.

Remember Rule #3 of arthritis management: Joints require movement to restore function and maintain optimal health. Medications don't replace this rule, but they can help you adhere to it. Let's begin with a discussion of the different medication options.

## TOPICAL PAIN MEDICATIONS

Topical pain relievers (analgesics) are applied to the skin over the part of the body that hurts. The active ingredient in the medication is absorbed through the skin to the site of pathology. As a group, these are perhaps the most underutilized medication alternative for arthritis. The primary advantage of topical medications is that they are usually the least invasive option because you don't ingest them, which decreases the risk of side effects. For example, topical capsaicin has been shown to be helpful when applied 4 times daily.

Consider all that has to happen for the painkilling ingredient in a swallowed pill to reach your sore joint(s). It reaches your stomach, where it is digested before being absorbed into your body in your intestines. The medication is now in your bloodstream, and will reach essentially all of the cells in your body, most of which do not need it. Finally, it must be broken down and metabolized by your liver and/or kidneys, and the resulting products of the breakdown excreted. This long journey can lead to a variety of systemic side effects, including injury to the stomach (a common problem), liver, and kidneys, as well as other parts of your body, depending on the medication ingredients. By contrast, a topical analgesic has minimal, if any, systemic absorption. It bypasses the digestive tract altogether.

Most topical pain relievers are available without a prescription. They can have many different ingredients. Their mechanism of action is an issue of some debate, and they may be underutilized because there has not been as much research about them as the other arthritis medications. Skeptics argue that very little of the active ingredient is actually absorbed through the skin, and that many topical solutions, including those that contain menthol, act by irritating the surrounding tissue, which increases blood flow to the joint or other painful area. This, in turn, would then presumably increase the elimination of inflammatory waste products.

Topical analgesics are available as creams, lotions, gels, and sprays. There are a few important points to consider if you decide to try one.

- ▶ Discuss this option with your doctor before using any analgesic; the fact that they are available without a prescription does not mean they are harmless.
- ▶ Purchase products that do not have an offensive odor and are not too messy. If it is unpleasant to use, chances are that you won't use it.
- ▶ Never place any topical medication over an open wound or sore.
- ▶ Buy products from reputable companies. Some over-the-counter topical analgesics have been found to have inert or even harmful substances.
- ▶ Wash your hands after using the topical agent to prevent accidental spreading to your mucous membranes, such as your eyes, nose, or mouth.

Topical analgesics are probably more effective for treating arthritis in peripheral joints, such as the fingers, wrists, elbows, and knees. However, they might also be worth trying if you have arthritis in your hips or other deeper joints.

Lidocaine is a potent topical medication that is available by pre-scription in a 5-percent patch. Lidocaine is similar to the novocaine used by dentists, and it acts by numbing the affected body part. It can be effective for arthritis of the knee and other peripheral joints, and it has few side effects. Each patch is used for 12 hours, with a 12-hour break before applying another patch. Some people find relief with this medication. Talk to your doctor about whether it might be right for you.

Basically, topical analgesics tend to have much lower rates of side effects and are well tolerated. They are a useful alternative if you require medication, and if using a topical analgesic can keep you from needing to take an oral drug,

## MEDICATIONS AVAILABLE WITHOUT A PRESCRIPTION

### Acetaminophen

Over-the-counter medications consist of two broad groups: anti-inflammatory and purely analgesic. Acetaminophen is primar-ily an analgesic medication that dulls the sensation of pain, al-though it probably reduces fever through an anti-inflammatory mechanism.

Acetaminophen does not help underlying inflammation in joints, but it can be a potent analgesic. It is generally well tolerated. No medication is without side effects, and acetaminophen is no exception. Only take acetaminophen as directed on the package. As discussed earlier, try one of the generics. If it doesn't work well enough, then try a brand-name product.

Acetaminophen is metabolized by the liver, and its potential side effects include liver damage. Do not drink alcohol when you are taking acetaminophen, as the combination can have serious effects on the liver. Overdoses of acetaminophen have occasion-ally been fatal, generally as the result of inadvertently combining them with other drugs or alcohol, or as the result of taking more than you realize. For example, many over-the-counter products contain acetaminophen, such as cold, headache, and sinus medications, so it is not uncommon to be taking more acetaminophen than you intended. Always read the active ingredients in any medication you take, and never take more than 4 grams of acetaminophen a day.

### Nonsteroidal Anti-inflammatory Drugs (NSAIDs)

Nonsteroidal anti-inflammatory medications (NSAIDs) include ibuprofen, indomethacin (Indocin®), nabumetone (Relafen®), and naproxen (Naprosyn®). Their mode of action differs from that of acetaminophen, because they affect the underlying inflammation as well as decrease pain. The main problem with these medications is their potential for side effects, which can include stomach pain, nausea, vomiting, diarrhea, stomach or intestinal ulceration and bleeding (sometimes in the absence of stomach pain), rash, ringing in the ears, kidney damage, and high blood pressure. Every year, an estimated 100,000–200,000 people are hospitalized due to side effects from NSAID use, and an estimated 10,000–20,000 deaths each year are believed to be related to NSAIDs. Aspirin is also an NSAID, but is rarely recommended because it has more side effects, especially when taken regularly, than newer medications.

Although they are sold over the counter in friendly looking boxes, NSAIDs are not benign medications. If you have high blood pressure or kidney problems, they are probably not the best choice for you. Nevertheless, they do have a place in the treatment of arthritis. If you are considering taking NSAIDs for long-term relief from the symptoms of arthritis, I strongly suggest that you try the recommendations in this book first, and also discuss the available treatment options with your personal physician.

NSAIDs and acetaminophen are sometimes taken together, because they work in different ways. It is my strong recommendation that you do this only on the advice of a physician. Otherwise, the risk of side effects outweighs the potential for gain.

## Prescription Medications

As with over-the-counter medications, the same two broad classes of prescription medications may be prescribed by your doctor for your arthritis: analgesics and anti-inflammatory medications.

Prescription analgesics include narcotic medications. They are potent painkillers, but they have major side effects, including drowsiness and constipation. Respiratory depression and a potential for abuse are also potentially serious complications. Before using narcotic medications to manage your arthritis, consider other options, such as injections, which will be discussed in the next chapter. Some prescription medications combine acetaminophen with a narcotic; others combine an NSAID with a narcotic. Discuss the different options with your doctor. Narcotic medications are commonly used during the acute period after surgery for arthritis.

Another prescription pain reliever is tramadol (Ultram®), which is similar in its mode of action to certain narcotics, in that it is an analgesic without anti-inflammatory effects. However, unlike narcotics, it does not depress respiration or have as great an addictive potential as narcotic medications. Side effects may include gastrointestinal upset, including pain, constipation, diarrhea, and vomiting, as well as dizziness, dry mouth, visual problems, and vertigo. Another medication in this class, Ultracet®, is a combination of acetaminophen and tramadol.

Prescription anti-inflammatory medications called *COX-2 inhibitors* have received a great deal of attention in recent years. As noted earlier, Bextra® and Vioxx® have been taken off the market due to serious side effects that outweigh their potential benefits. Celebrex® (celecoxib) is still available, but it is prescribed much less frequently than it used to be.

The basic mechanism of action of the COX-2 inhibitors is similar to that of NSAIDs. Traditional NSAIDs block two enzymes, COX-1 and COX-2. The COX-2 enzyme is the one that needs to be blocked in order to inhibit inflammation. Unfortunately, the lining of the stomach can be damaged when the COX-1 enzyme is also blocked. There is also the potential for kidney damage and high blood pressure when the COX-1 enzyme is blocked. Initially, it was believed that selectively blocking the COX-2 enzyme would diminish these side effects. In addition, because the COX-1 enzyme would not be blocked, it would be possible to take a higher dosage of the COX-2 blocker, and thus achieve greater control of inflammation and pain. This worked well in laboratory studies, and also in early human studies.

Celebrex® sometimes causes indigestion, diarrhea, and abdominal discomfort. It can also have serious side effects, such as skin reactions, bleeding, kidney damage, stroke, and heart problems. Still, Celebrex® may be a good option for some people. If you have not been able to control your arthritis pain and inflammation with other medications, discuss Celebrex® with your physician.

# 22

# Injections

IN ADDITION to topical and oral medications, drugs can be injected directly into affected joints. One general benefit of injection is that the effect is more localized and less systemic, and it provides a greater concentration of the active ingredient of a medication directly to the damaged tissue. A general negative is that any injection carries certain risks, including infection, bleeding, and adverse reaction to the medication.

There is no magic bullet that will take away your symptoms and reverse your arthritis, but injections can provide significant pain relief. It is important that you not squander this relief. Injection therapy should be considered as just one component of a comprehensive treatment approach that includes participating in structured physical therapy exercises and making appropriate diet and supplement choices.

The two substances commonly injected into joints to treat arthritis are steroids and hyaluronic acid.

## STEROID INJECTIONS

Steroids are potent anti-inflammatory medications. A steroid injection directly into a joint is often very effective in temporarily controlling symptoms when a joint becomes acutely symptomatic from a flare-up of arthritis and more conservative measures have failed to control the symptoms.

Steroid injections tend to adhere to the law of diminishing returns. The first one is often quite effective, and symptoms may be relieved for 3–4 months. Subsequent injections tend to be less effective. Most physicians will only inject a single joint 3–4 times in a 2-year period, because steroids can *cause* further deterioration of the joint and surrounding structures. Of course, each person must be treated individually; steroids are not an appropriate treatment for everyone.

The steroid in the injection is generally mixed with an anesthetic. Depending on the anatomy of your joint and the skill of your physician, steroid injections can be a bit painful. The injection itself should not take more than a few minutes. Depending on the joint being injected, your doctor may use an imaging technique, such as an X-ray or ultrasound, to help guide the needle and make certain that the tip is in the right place when the medication is injected.

Take it easy after an injection for the rest of the day, and don't do more than a bit of light walking if the injection was in a weight-bearing joint. After the injection, the joint might feel numb, and the pain can return when the anesthetic wears off. It may take 3–5 days to experience the steroid's maximum effect, although everyone responds differently.

To prevent infection, your physician needs to maintain sterile conditions during the procedure. Rarely, a joint can have a "post-injection flare" in which symptoms temporarily worsen. The flare will generally subside within 48–72 hours. If this happens to you, call your doctor for further care, and also to help rule out an infection. In addition to the effects on the joint, steroid injections can raise blood sugar levels, so people with diabetes need to be especially aware of this potential side effect and discuss it with their doctor. A steroid injection can change the pigmentation of the skin, making it lighter. This is a rare complication, but it is a potential problem, particularly in people with darker skin. There are other side effects, and some people are not good candidates for steroid injections. If you are taking a blood thinner, you may need to discontinue it prior to the injection. It is important to discuss the potential benefits and risks with your physician. If you do have a steroid injection, be sure to have it done by a qualified, experienced professional.

As with the other treatment options discussed above, any symptom relief gained from an injection is temporary, and this period of relief should be seen as a "window of opportunity," during which you can participate more fully in a structured physical therapy program. The symptom relief achieved from an injection can hopefully be maintained and even improved upon with exercise, in conjunction with appropriate diet and supplements. Do not start exercising until at least 1 day after an injection. Symptom relief can take 3–5 days, or even longer, so it may be a week or more before you are ready for physical therapy.

## Hyaluronic Acid

Another effective procedure is to inject hyaluronic acid directly into the joint. This is done most commonly in the knee, but it has also been used in other joints, including the hip and shoulder. As discussed earlier, each mobile joint in the body consists of a joint capsule made of tough fibrous tissue that connects the two bones of the joint. The synovium lines the inside of the joint capsule and secretes thick, viscous synovial fluid. This fluid and water are the chief components of joint fluid. The important viscous quality is due in large part to the presence of hyaluronic acid.

Hyaluronic acid provides nourishment to the cartilage and helps remove waste products. It also provides lubrication for the shear stresses (side-to-side forces) on the joint, acts as a shock absorber, and lubricates and potentially shields the pain receptors that line the joint.

Hyaluronic acid levels are decreased in an arthritic joint, and injecting it into a joint increases the levels of hyaluronic acid within the joint, and may even stimulate cartilage growth. It is still not completely clear how injections of hyaluronic acid help relieve the symptoms of arthritis, because the hyaluronic acid in the injection remains there for a period of only days, while symptom relief may last for months. What does seem clear is that the injections do help a significant number of people. Patients with mild-to-moderate arthritis receive the most benefit from hyaluronic acid injections. It is less likely to be helpful once arthritis has become severe and the joint anatomy is basically bone on bone, with little cartilage or joint space left.

As with steroid injections, some people report immediate relief from a single injection of hyaluronic acid. Others may require a series of 3 or more injections, given a week apart, before experiencing symptom relief. When pain relief is achieved, it may last for as long as 3–12 months.

There are currently five FDA-approved injectable preparations of hyaluronic acid: Synvisc®, Hyalgan®, Supartz®, Orthovisc®, and Euflexxa®. Some are given as a series of five injections; others require only three. Whether or not you receive benefit from the first injection, the entire series is typically given because the effect can be cumulative. Synvisc® was the first hyaluronic acid preparation available in the United States, and many physicians use it or the next formulation that was approved, Hyalgan®. The disadvantage of Synvisc® is a slightly increased possibility of creating a reactive flare. When this occurs, the joint becomes inflamed, and a steroid injection is needed to reduce the inflammation. None of the hyaluronic acid preparations has been proven superior to the others.

Most of the research on hyaluronic acid injections has been for arthritis of the knee, and this is the condition for which it has received FDA approval. However, many physicians use it for other joints, including the hip, shoulder, ankle, and first carpometacarpal joint in the hand; research for its efficacy in joints other than the knee is ongoing. X-ray or ultrasound guidance for placement of the injection should be used in joints other than the knee. Many physicians believe that an injection into the knee is not technically challenging enough to warrant the use of image-guidance; others argue that ultrasound or X-ray guidance should be used for all intra-articular injections.

As noted previously for steroid injections and medications, hyaluronic acid injections may help with the symptoms of arthritis but they are not a cure. Their use should be seen as a window of opportunity during which time you can participate in a structured physical therapy program.

# 23

# Surgical Options

I ALWAYS TELL my patients the only thing you can't do after surgery is change your mind—once you have surgery there is no
going back. Although surgery is generally considered as a last re-
sort, it can be an effective treatment for certain cases of arthritis.
The four main kinds of surgery for arthritis are arthroscopic repair,
osteotomy, arthrodesis, and total joint arthroplasty.

*Arthroscopy* is the least invasive procedure. It involves making
minimal incisions in the skin and inserting a small arthroscope
(basically a camera) into the joint. Using small instruments, the
surgeon removes the damaged parts of the joint and cleans it. Clean-
ing the joint may involve removing fragments of bone or cartilage,
removing inflamed synovial tissue, trimming and smoothing torn
articular cartilage, and repairing any torn meniscus in the knee.
Arthroscopy can temporarily relieve the symptoms of arthritis of
the hip and knee.

The risks of arthroscopy include rare complications of anesthesia. Doing the procedure under local anesthesia helps to minimize
this problem. Other risks include bleeding, infection, nerve damage, and scarring. The recovery period after arthroscopy is variable,
but generally involves several weeks of rehabilitation.

An *osteotomy* is performed when arthritis has damaged one specific area of bone. In this procedure, a piece (or pieces) of bone is

removed from the joint in order to realign it. This procedure is appropriate for younger, active patients with preserved functional joint range of motion, a small joint malalignment that needs correcting, and/or pathology that is restricted to one portion of the joint. If a joint malalignment is contributing to the progression of arthritis, correcting the malalignment and removing the diseased portion of bone may reduce symptoms, redistribute the weight to the healthy part of the joint, and slow progression of the arthritis. Risks of an osteotomy are rare, but include complications of anesthesia, infection, bleeding, nerve damage, and scarring.

An *arthrodesis* is a fusion of the joint. The use of this type of procedure for an arthritic joint has been declining, and it is used in only selected cases. However, it may be indicated for some people who are older and have arthritis confined to one joint with good preservation of the surrounding tissues. Some joints, such as those in the ankle, foot, hand, and wrist, may be appropriately treated with arthrodesis. Risks and potential complications include the complications of anesthesia, pain at the fusion site, failure of the fusion, bleeding, infection, nerve injury, and damage to the neighboring joints because their biomechanics were altered by the fusion.

The most invasive surgical procedure for joint arthritis is a total joint *arthroplasty*. This is the technical term for total joint replacement, in which the entire joint is removed and a prosthetic one is inserted. Replacement surgery is not possible for all joints. They are most common in the hip and knee, but shoulder joint and other joint replacement surgeries are also gaining popularity. Total joint replacement has seen increasing use as the procedure has become more technically advanced and successful.

## Hip and Knee Replacement

There are different types of prostheses, with different features, and you can discuss the options with your doctor. A hip replacement can be performed using either a cement or non-cement type of glue. A cemented prosthesis allows the patient to return to full weight-bearing activities sooner than a non-cemented one. With a non-cemented hip prosthesis, it may be 3 months or longer before the patient can put all of her weight on the affected limb. However, a non-cemented prosthesis is ultimately stronger, and may be easier to deal with than a cemented prosthesis if additional surgery is ever required. In general, an older, less active patient who will probably not wear through it is offered a cemented hip prosthesis, while a younger, more active patient is typically offered the non-cemented one. Cemented prostheses are typically used in knee replacements.

When performed on the appropriate patients, total knee or hip replacement surgery is often very effective in reducing symptoms and returning people with arthritis to an active lifestyle. As with any surgery, however, there are risks and potential complications. Risks can include complications of anesthesia, infection, bleeding, and nerve damage, but are rare when procedures are performed by an experienced surgeon. Another major potential complication is that a blood clot, called a deep venous thrombosis (DVT), may form after the procedure. A pulmonary embolus (PE) can occur if this clot breaks away and circulates in the bloodstream. This can lead to death. If blood thinners are not given after surgery, a significant number of people with a hip or knee replacement may develop such a clot. If you are not a candidate for blood-thinning medication, a filter can be placed in one of the veins leading to the heart to trap any clots that form and break away, so there will be less of a chance a clot will be carried to your lungs.

Another risk is that the prosthesis can malfunction or move out of position. Part of your discussion with your doctor about the risks, potential complications, and alternative treatments should include a discussion about your postoperative rehabilitation care, including any medications such as blood thinners, and how long you will need to take them, so you will know what to expect and be prepared.

A *hemiarthroplasty* is another surgical option. In contrast to a total arthroplasty, a hemiarthroplasty replaces only part of the joint. In some joints, such as the shoulder, hemiarthroplasty is generally preferable to total joint arthroplasty.

## GET A SECOND OPINION

Before having surgery, get a second opinion. People are often hesitant to get second opinions, but they shouldn't be. A good doctor does not mind when his patients get another opinion. Probably both doctors will agree with the chosen course of action, but what if they don't? You owe it to yourself to find out if different doctors have different opinions about your best course of action, particularly before you undergo a major operation

Remember the fourth rule of arthritis management: Treat the patient, not the X-ray. If your doctor tells you that you need an operation because your X-ray indicates you have severe arthritis, get another opinion. Surgery should be reserved for significant symptoms that interfere with quality of life and that have been resistant to aggressive, conservative care that included exercise, diet, supplementation, medications, and injections.

If you and your doctor decide that surgery is the right option, you still need to follow the principles outlined in this book. Take as good care of yourself as possible before surgery. Exercising, eating right, and taking appropriate supplements will help maximize your chances of success after surgery. Talk to your surgeon about the supplements you are taking. He may ask you to discontinue taking omega-3 fatty acids, because they can thin the blood. Exercise will help keep the surrounding muscles fit and ready for action during rehabilitation. Sticking with a healthy diet and taking supplements will help you to continue to exercise, and will also help keep the rest of your joints healthy.

## QUESTIONS TO ASK YOUR SURGEON BEFORE SURGERY

- What are the risks and potential complications of this procedure?

- How many of these procedures have you done?

- How would you define a successful operation for this procedure? Will I be pain-free after the procedure?

- What is your success rate for this procedure?

- What complications have you seen with this procedure?

- What is your complication rate for this procedure? How does your complication rate compare with other doctors?

- What alternative treatments are available?

- If I have one of the alternative treatments and it doesn't work, can I still get this surgery later?

- If I have this surgery now, can I still have the other treatments later? Does this surgery close the door to other kinds of treatment?

- If it were you in my situation, would you have this procedure done?

- If you were having this procedure done, which doctor would you choose to do it? Can I have his or her number so I can get a second opinion?

- How long is the recovery process?

- What will the recovery process involve?

- When will I be able to go back to work and exercise?

# 24.

## Conclusion

D UE DILIGENCE refers to the process of gathering all the information that could reasonably have an effect on a transaction we are considering. Before buying a car, for example, we investigate the quality of the brand, the reputation of the dealer, and the desirability of the other cars available at comparable prices.

Due diligence is just as important to your health as it is to your wallet. If you have joint pain, make sure you receive the best possible treatment. Even if you don't have joint pain, you should try to stay healthy to prevent future problems.

As we have seen, the symptoms of arthritis can often be controlled and eliminated through a combination of nutrition, exercise, and supplementation. Along the way, by taking care of your arthritis, you will also be taking care of your entire body. It's a worthwhile investment, perhaps the most important one you can make.

I hope you have enjoyed reading this book, and that you will use the information to start making healthy lifestyle changes. You don't need me to tell you how important it is to stay healthy. It's one of those things we all know is important, but our daily choices don't always reflect this understanding. By reading this book you have already demonstrated that you are motivated and interested in improving your joint health. As we have seen, identifying good health as one of your core values will help you to stay motivated.

The choices you make on a daily basis will become a simple manifestation of this value. Your choices will soon become good, healthy habits. You may have joint pain today, but that doesn't mean you will always have joint pain.

As you make lifestyle changes, remember to start small. Your small changes will add up, and soon they will become big changes that feel natural and leave you feeling great. Don't stop your learning with this book. Continue to gather information from a variety of sources. Learning is a lifelong journey. No one can take as good care of your body as you can. Take what you have learned from this book and talk with your friends, family, and doctors.

I wish you all the best with your current and future endeavors. And I wish you good health, because with health all things are possible.

# Glossary

Alpha-linolenic acid – An essential omega-3 fatty acid that is a component of many common vegetable oils.

Arthrodesis – The surgical fusion of a joint.

Arthroscopy – A minimally invasive surgical procedure in which damage to the interior of a joint is visualized using an arthroscope, which is inserted into the joint through one small incision while surgical instruments are inserted through another.

Antioxidants – Molecules that can slow or prevent the oxidation of other molecules and thereby reduce the production of free radicals and prevent damage to cells.

Arthritis – A joint problem that involves inflammation, pain, and/or stiffness.

Autoimmune disease – Any disease that results from an abnormal immune response that involves failure of an organism to recognize one of its constituent parts—such as components of a joint—as "self."

Bioavailability – The amount of an ingested food that is actually absorbed by the body.

Body biomechanics – The study of how skeletal structures function together in space under the influence of gravity and other forces.

Bone spur –Also known as *osteophytes*, they are bony projections that form on and in joints. Bone spurs form in response to increased pressure placed on joints, most often as the result of arthritis. They may limit joint movement and cause pain.

Bursa – A small, fluid-filled sac located at the point where a muscle or tendon slides across bone, reducing friction between the two moving surfaces.

Cartilage – A tough, flexible connective tissue that provides lubrication as well as shock-absorbing function for mobile joints.

Carotenoids – Antioxidant compounds that occur naturally in plants and give fruits and vegetables their bright color.

Chondrocytes – The cells within a joint that make cartilage.

Chondroitin – Negatively charged molecules within cartilage that provide strong cushioning for the joint by repelling each other when a joint is stressed (such as during weight-bearing).

Collagen – A fibrous protein that has great tensile strength, and is the main component of fascia, cartilage, ligaments, tendons, and bone.

Computed tomography (CT) – A medical imaging method that generates a three-dimensional image of the internal structure of a joint or other tissue from a large series of two-dimensional X-ray images.

Docosahexaenoic acid (DHA) – An omega-3 fatty acid most often found in fish oil.

Eicosapentaenoic acid (EHA) – An omega-3 fatty acid that is a metabolite of alpha-linolenic acid.

Electrocardiogram (EKG) – A test that examines the electrical conduction of the heart to help determine the health of the heart tissue and its electrical conductivity.

Fixed joint – A joint whose component bones do not move, as with the bones of the skull.

Flexible joint – A joint that is movable, such as the hip or shoulder.

Flexibility – The range of motion at a given joint.

Gamma-linolenic acid (GLA) – An omega-3 fatty acid found in evening primrose seed oil, borage seed oil, and flaxseed oil.

Glucosamine – An "amino sugar" that helps cartilage hold water; may enable the joint to produce more cartilage.

Hyaluronic acid – A component of joint fluid that helps to lubricate and cushion the joint.

Hydrogenation – This process converts an oil into a solid; it extends the shelf life of foods but the trans fats produced are believed to contribute to heart disease.

Hydrophilic – Accepting of water; dissolves more readily in water than in oil.

Hydrophobic – Rejecting of water; not soluble in water.

Inflammation – A complex biological response by the body to harmful stimuli, including bacteria, viruses, fungus, irritants, and physical injury. Chronic inflammation can lead to a number of diseases, including arthritis.

International unit (IU) – The amount of a given substance that is based on the biological activity required to produce a given effect; a way to standardize the amount of vitamins, mineral, or other substances, without simply relying on weight.

Joint – The location at which two or more bones make contact. Joints are constructed to allow movement and provide mechanical support.

Ligament – Tough fibrous bands of tissue that attach bones to other bones, providing support and strength to joints.

Linoleic acid – An essential omega-6 fatty acid that is abundant in many vegetable oils, especially safflower and sunflower oils.

Magnetic resonance imaging (MRI) – An imaging test that is often optimal to evaluate the soft tissues of the body and uses radio waves and magnetic fields, not radiation.

Muscle – A group of individual muscle fibers that combine to form larger bundles that collectively contract and relax to move the body through space.

Negative phase – That portion of an exercise repetition when the muscle is elongating (lengthening).

Neuromodulator – A substance other than a neurotransmitter, released by a neuron at a synapse and conveying information to a region of neurons, either enhancing or dampening their activities.

Neurotransmitter – Chemicals that are used to relay, amplify, and modulate electrical signals between a neuron and another cell.

Nerve – An enclosed, cable-like bundle of axons (the long, slender projection of a neuron) that transmits information from the bodies of neurons to distant cells.

Nociceptive nerve – A nerve that is capable of communicating pain and that is part of the nervous system's pain pathways that communicate painful stimuli to the brain.

Omega-3 fatty acids – A family of polyunsaturated fatty acids that are found in the membranes of cells and that make them more flexible and pliable. Important omega-3 fatty acids in nutrition include alpha-linolenic acid (ALA), eicosapentaenoic acid (EPA), and docosahexaenoic acid (DHA). Omega-3 fatty acids have an anti-inflammatory effect on the body

Omega-6 fatty acids – Fatty acids that are found in the membranes of cells and that tend to make them less flexible and pliable. Omega-6 fatty acids have a proinflammatory effect on the body when the ratio of omega-6 to omega-3 is too high.

Omega-9 fatty acids – A class of unsaturated fatty acids that can be produced from unsaturated fat and that are therefore not considered "essential" fatty acids. Mediterranean diets have a high level of omega-9 fatty acids.

Oleic acid – A monounsaturated omega-9 fatty acid found in various animal and vegetable sources; olive oil is an especially rich source of oleic acid.

Orthotics – The science of developing equipment that supports and stabilizes a part of the body that is weak or malformed. An *orthosis* is a mechanical device that is applied to or around a part of the body in order to optimize function and/or help restore and/or maintain optimal body biomechanics. For example, they can increase stability in an unstable joint and prevent a deformed foot from developing additional problems. One example of a foot orthosis is an arch support.

Osteoarthritis – The most common form of arthritis, a condition also known as *degenerative arthritis* or *degenerative joint disease*. It is the wearing of the cartilage that covers and acts as a cushion inside joints; symptoms may include pain, stiffness, and/or inflammation.

Osteophyte – An abnormal bone overgrowth. See "Bone spur."

Osteoporosis – A disease of bone in which bone mineral density is decreased, leading to an increased risk of fracture.

Osteotomy – A surgical procedure in which bone is cut to shorten, lengthen, or change its alignment. It is one method to relieve pain in arthritis, especially of the hip and knee.

Oxidative response – The production of free radicals that can attack foreign invaders such as viruses or bacteria, but that can also damage the body's own healthy tissue.

Oxygen Radical Absorbance Capacity (ORAC) – A laboratory test developed by the United States government to measure the antioxidant capacity of fruits, vegetables, and other foods.

Parasympathetic nervous system – The part of the nervous system that is active when you are resting and digesting. It participates in the process of digesting your food, slowing your heart rate and lowering your blood pressure.

Polyphenols – Powerful antioxidants found in plants.

Positive phase – The portion of a repetition in a given exercise characterized by the muscle contracting.

Primary osteoarthritis – This form of arthritis tends to occur after age 45; no identifiable cause of cartilage degradation is evident. A combination of genetic predisposition and normal "wear and tear" of the joints from repetitive microtrauma may contribute to its development.

Proprioceptive nerve – This type of nerves communicates position sense from the body to the brain.

Proteoglycans – Core proteins attached to carbohydrate chains that are one of the important building blocks of cartilage.

Repetition – A single movement through a given exercise in strength training.

Rheumatoid arthritis – An autoimmune arthritis in which the body's immune system attacks the synovium in the joint capsule.

Slightly flexible joints – This type of joint is only slightly mobile, such as the joints between the vertebrae and the sacroiliac joints.

Sclerosis – A condition that involves hardening of tissue. In osteoarthritis, it refers to hardening of the bone.

Secondary osteoarthritis – A type of arthritis in which an identifiable event, such as a severe trauma or repetitive microtrauma, triggers degradation of the cartilage.

Subchondral cyst – A fluid-filled pocket beneath the bone that may form in osteoarthritis. It may be accompanies by joint-space narrowing and sclerosis.

Sympathetic nervous system – The part of the nervous system that is responsible for regulating many of the body's basic mechanisms, ranging from pupil diameter and gut motility to the "fight or flight" response.

Synovium – The soft tissue that lines the non-cartilaginous surfaces within joint cavities and secretes synovial fluid.

Synovial fluid – A thick, straw-colored fluid within the joint that is secreted by the cells of the synovium.

Synovial joint – Each synovial joint has the same basic structure, including an outer joint capsule, synovium lining the capsule, synovial fluid, cartilage, and articulating bones.

Systemic illness – An illness in which the entire body is affected rather than a single organ or part of the body.

Tendon – A tough band of connective tissue that attaches muscle to bone and is built to withstand tension.

Topical medication – A medication that is applied to the skin.

Total joint arthroplasty – A total joint replacement.

Type I muscle fiber – Slow-twitch, small muscle fibers used for carrying light loads over long distances. These fibers have increased resistance to fatigue, and are well suited for activities related to physical effort requiring strength and endurance.

Type II muscle fiber – Fast-twitch, large muscle fibers used for lifting heavy loads. They are less suited to continuous types of activity and are more suited to rapid alternating effort.

X-ray – An imaging technique that utilizes electromagnetic radiation, primarily used to visualize bony structures.

# Web Sites for Further Information

http://www.arthritis.org/
The homepage for the Arthritis Foundation
The Arthritis Foundation is a voluntary not-for-profit organization that supports more than 100 types of arthritis and related conditions with advocacy programs, services, and research.

http://www.niams.nih.gov/hi/topics/arthritis/oahandout.htm
http://www.niams.nih.gov/hi/topics/arthritis/oahandout.htm
This Web site is offered by the National Institute of Arthritis and Musculo-skeletal and Skin Diseases (NIAMS) and the National Institutes of Health (NIH). It covers a wide range of issues relating to osteoarthritis.

http://www.hopkins-arthritis.org/
This is a Web site from Johns Hopkins Medicine that includes informa-tion on all types of arthritis, including treatments.

http://www.mayoclinic.com/health/osteoarthritis/DS00019
This Web site from the Mayo clinic offers a good basic overview and review of osteoarthritis.

http://www.medicinenet.com/osteoarthritis/article.htm
This Web site provides a good overview of osteoarthritis, its causes, and treatment strategies.

http://www.nlm.nih.gov/medlineplus/osteoarthritis.html
MedLine Plus is a service of the National Library of Medicine and the

National Institutes of Health (NIH). This Web site offers a wide range of articles related to osteoarthritis, as well as links to specific osteoarthritis conditions; for example, arthritis of the base of the thumb.

http://www.emedicinehealth.com/osteoarthritis/article_em.htm
This eMedicineHealth.com article provides a good overview of osteo-arthritis

http://www.rheumatology.org/public/factsheets/oa_new.asp
This is an informational Web site about osteoarthritis offered by the American College of Rheumatology.

http://orthopedics.about.com/cs/arthritis/a/arthritis.htm
This is an informational Web site about osteoarthritis with several links to more specific forms of arthritis and its treatments.

http://www.aapmr.org/condtreat/pain/arthritis.htm
This is an informational Web site about arthritis provided by the American Academy of Physical Medicine and Rehabilitation.

# Additional Reading

*Arthritis: A Take Care of Yourself Health Guide* by James F. Fries. New York: Perseus Books, 1999.

*Arthritis for Dummies* by Sarah Brewer. New York: Wiley, 2004.

*The Arthritis Helpbook: A Tested Self-Management Program for Coping with Arthritis and Fibromyalgia, 5th Edition* by Kate Lorig and James F. Fries. New York: Harper Collins, 2000.

*The Arthritis Cure: The Medical Miracle That Can Halt, Reverse, and May Even Cure Osteoarthritis* by Jason Theodosakis and Sheila Buff. New York: Saint Martin's Paperbacks, 2003.

*Strong Women and Men Beat Arthritis* by Miriam E. Nelson. New York: Putnam Adult, 2002.

*Living SMART: Five Essential Skills to Change Your Health Habits Forever* by Joshua C. Klapow, PhD and Sheri D. Pruitt, PhD. New York: DiaMedica, 2008.

# Index

Note: **Boldface** numbers indicate illustrations and tables.